About the author

Jane Sarasohn-Kahn is a health economist, advisor, and trend weaver to organizations focused at the intersection of health, technology and people – especially consumers, patients and caregivers. Jane's consultancy THINK-Health collaborates with stakeholders spanning the health/care ecosystem.

Jane sits on many advisory boards in health technology, patient advocacy, and health media. She is also on the board of The Clinic, a free clinic in Phoenixville, Pennsylvania. Jane is a frequent speaker and prolific writer, founding the *Health Populi* blog in 2007. Jane has also contributed to the Huffington Post, Tincture on Medium, the Washington Post Health Care Rx panel and other publications.

Jane has received many kudos in social media: among them, being one of the Top 100 Most Influential Economists in the World, a Top Twitter Account to Follow in Digital Health, One of the #HIT100, and one of Rock Health's Women in Healthcare.

Jane holds an MA (Economics) and MHSA (Health Policy) from the University of Michigan. While Jane loves her work, she is even more passionate about family and home, Slow Food and her local CSA, and living a full life. Jane tweets @HealthyThinker on Twitter and hosts her websites on www.healthpopuli.com and www.janesarasohnkahn.com

HealthConsuming™
From health consumer to health citizen

Jane Sarasohn-Kahn

Published in May 2019, by

Jane Sarasohn-Kahn MA (Econ.), MHSA
Health Economist, Advisor, Trend Weaver
www.healthpopuli.com

ISBN: 978-0-578-48139-5

Designed and Illustrated by
Flat World Technology
Philadelphia

Printed by
Brilliant Graphics
Exton, Pennsylvania

Fonts
Bebas Neue and Museo Sans 300

Author photo by Joe Shields

Acknowledgements

I thank and appreciate so many people who have shaped my perspectives on health, healthcare and living well. In the beginning, there were two parents who surrounded me with love and the best education possible. Charles and Polly Sarasohn were the most important social determinants of health in my life. They also, each in their unique ways, showed me the power of an engaged patient. My mother died too young, succumbing to a rare form of leukemia but surviving eight years beyond her six-month-survival prognosis powered by the active role she played in her medical and self-care. My father, based on smart lifestyle choices and access to great medical services, lived well and long, dying at a ripe old age, a bionic man by then.

The first person to recommend I enroll in an economics course at the University of Michigan was Jeffrey Sachs; without his urging, I would never have signed up for ECON 101. Thereafter, William Neenan SJ connected the dots between economics, politics, and Everyday People, and then at the U-M School of Public Health, Irene Butter and Ken Warner bolstered my interest in cost-effectiveness analysis with a hard head and a soft heart. Professors Gary Becker at the University of Chicago and Uwe Reinhardt of Princeton University were impactful teachers.

Anne Wright hired and brought me to Philadelphia after grad school, and we worked in health consulting across America to help hospitals manage, grow and adopt new technologies and services. I expanded my geographic horizons and challenged my learning curve in London, where I worked with the health care team at Touche Ross, in and beyond the National Health Service and the UK. On the continent, Jean-Claude Healy at WHO was my first teacher on eHealth at the very beginning.

The health care team at Institute for the Future taught me how to read health-tech tea leaves: I thank my mentors Ian Morrison and Wendy Everett and my longtime colleague Matthew Holt with whom I share both love of Chelsea football and health policy wonkiness.

Eric Topol, MD, Joseph Kvedar MD, Harm Scherpbier, MD, and Prof. Dr. Koen Kas are my digital health touchpoints, keeping me practically smart, humble and hopeful.

Juhan Sonin first taught me about the importance of design for making information beautiful. Eric Karten did the same for helping me get how design can enchant medical products.

The Ladies Who Dine keep me grounded, laughing and smart: Alexandra Drane, Susannah Fox, Margaret Laws, and Lisa Suennen – I raise my champagne glass to you.

I am grateful that Brian Klepper and Michael Millenson challenge me, even when I know what I think I know. Appreciation to many who shared wisdom reviewing the *HealthConsuming* drafts: along with Harm, Lisa and Matthew, Emily Hackel Reitz, Reavis Hilz-Ward, Deven McGraw, and Lygeia Ricciardi provided invaluable input.

John Enyart of Flat World Technology, and Karl Mooney, designer-and-book-whisperer – there's no *HealthConsuming* without you two on my team.

I thank my clients, who span all aspects of health. My only profession since leaving U-M Ann Arbor has been advising organizations serving health and healthcare, both in large consulting firms and via THINK-Health, my consultancy. I've collaborated with some of my clients for years; many of you have become dear friends. I value these relationships, where I learn at least as much from you as you do from me.

Finally, Robert and Anna Kahn remind me, every day, that love is the ultimate vitamin.

Phoenixville, PA
March 2019

HealthConsuming™

What if ... people got a fair ROI for healthcare spending the way we expect a reasonable return from other investments?

Chapter 1

WE ARE ALL HEALTH CONSUMERS NOW

"The need for action now is clear. Health care costs are climbing so fast they may soon threaten the quality of care and access to care which Americans enjoy." Ronald Reagan said this in 1983. In the U.S. then, health care costs were rising three times the rate of inflation. President Reagan noted that health care costs were consuming a growing portion of the U.S. gross domestic product: 10.5 percent of GDP in 1982, compared with 5.9 percent in 1965. [1]

Nearly fifty years later, it's *déjà vu* all over again.

In 2018, most Americans said that health care was the top public policy issue, ahead of taxes, immigration, the environment, and education. [2] It wasn't just consumer-voters that were keen to address health care reform, and especially health care costs. The American Hospital Association and America's Health Insurance Plans (AHIP), the health insurance association, publicly advocated for health care reform, and especially to lower the cost of prescription drugs, in an op-ed titled, "When your medication costs more than your mortgage." [3]

As he was preparing to exit the Cleveland Clinic as CEO, Dr. Toby Cosgrove was interviewed by CNBC's "Power Lunch" program and said, "the rising cost of U.S. health care is a huge threat to the U.S. economy," noting that 20 percent of hospitals were running in the red.[4]

Health care costs were a "tapeworm eating at our economic body," Warren Buffett observed in 2010.[5]

The Mayo Clinic has been named one of the best hospitals in the United States by *Consumer Reports*, HealthGrades, and *U.S. News and World Reports*. In March 2017, a story appeared in the *Minneapolis Star-Tribune* titled, "Mayo to give preference to privately insured patients over Medicaid patients."[6] In this article, Dr. John Noseworthy, Mayo Clinic's Chief Executive Officer, was quoted discussing the growing share of patients covered by Medicaid that were served by the hospital. Dr. Noseworthy noted that Medicaid reimbursement covered 50 to 85 cents on every dollar charged by the hospital.

"We're asking ... if the patient has commercial insurance, or they're Medicaid or Medicare patients and they're equal, that we prioritize the commercial insured patients enough so ... we can be financially strong at the end of the year to continue to advance our mission," Dr. Noseworthy said.

A few days after the *Tribune* published this article, the Mayo Clinic's communications department issued a statement: "Patient medical need will always be the primary factor in determining and setting an appointment....Changing demographics, aging of Americans and budgetary pressures at state and federal government pose challenges to the fiscal sustainability in health care today," Dr. Noseworthy explained.[7]

That's the stark reality of health care in America at one of the top medical centers in the country and, indeed, the world.

The United States spends more on health care, and more per person, than any other nation on the planet. U.S. health care spending reached $3.7 trillion in 2018 – about $11,200 per person. Health care spending is approaching nearly one-fifth of the U.S. gross domestic product. That's $1 in every $5 in the national economy. By 2026, national health expenditures will reach $5.7 trillion – over $16,000 *per capita*.[8]

Consider America's high spending on health care with the sobering fact that, for the first time since 1993, life expectancy in the United States declined in 2016.[9] Life expectancy in the U.S. used to be one year above the OECD average in 1970. In 2017, it was two years *below* the OECD average.[10]

The U.S. gets a low return-on-investment (ROI) for its exorbitant spending on health care, the Organisation for Economic Co-operation and Development (OECD) has noted for several years in the annual report on member nations' health care systems. The 2018 analysis included special U.S. country notes asking, "How does the United States compare?" with its sister OECD countries. Across most population health, access, and mortality measures, the answer was, "Not well."

The sad economic arithmetic works out to be, "spend more, get (much) less." Specifically, the U.S. spends much more, and for that huge investment achieves epidemic levels of obesity and poor access to health care services for its residents.

On the measure of lifespan, here are the facts on the return on investment for health care spending. The OECD average spending

PEER COUNTRIES GENERATED GREATER HEALTH GAINS THAN THE UNITED STATES, WHILE THE RATE OF GROWTH IN HEALTHCARE'S SHARE OF GDP WAS SIMILAR

Percentage change in life expectancy, disease burden, and health spending as a share of GDP, 1991-2016

■ United States   ■ Comparable Country Average

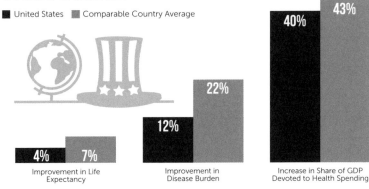

| Improvement in Life Expectancy | Improvement in Disease Burden | Increase in Share of GDP Devoted to Health Spending |

4% 7%   12% 22%   40% 43%

Source: Kaiser Family Foundation analysis of data from OECD, Institute for Health Metrics and Evaluation, and National Health Expenditure (NHE) data from Centers for Medicare and Medicaid Services.

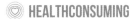 HEALTHCONSUMING

for health care was $4,069 *per capita/citizen* in 2017. The U.S. spent about two-and-one-half-times that, $10,209, followed by Switzerland which spent $8,009 and Luxembourg at $6,475. The Swiss life expectancy at birth in 2017 was 83.7 years, and for Luxembourg, 82.8 years.

American life expectancy in 2017 was 78.6 years.[11]

Both Switzerland and Luxembourg have a form of universal health coverage, with compulsory social insurance. The United States does not ensure universal health care. Citizens and legislators are locked in a struggle about whether access to health insurance should be rolled back from the inadequate place it currently stands.

In the U.S., many social determinants have contributed to a life expectancy reversal since 2016. One tragic contributor to higher mortality at younger age is the growing rates of death from suicide, accidents and drug overdoses, termed "deaths of despair" by Princeton University professors Anne Case and Angus Deaton. "You can find episodes like the flu epidemic or wartimes when mortality rates go up, but sustained increases in mortality for any major group in any society are really quite rare. It's an indication that something is very wrong," their research revealed.[12]

The high rate of obesity in the U.S. also contributes to reducing life expectancy in America. Obesity led to nearly 200,000 "excess deaths" in 2011 and reduced life expectancy by nearly one year at age 40. Deaths due to heart disease consistently declined for nearly 40 years, but began to tick up in 2014 as obesity rates climbed, contributing to type 2 diabetes, sleep apnea, and cancer.[13]

At the same time, health care costs have become the top pocketbook issue for most Americans, above concerns about how to pay for food, housing, and utilities.[14] Middle-class household spending on health care in the U.S. increased by 25 percent between 2007 and 2014, while spending on basic needs — food at home, housing, transportation, and clothing — fell during that period.[15]

A dramatic risk-shift occurred in the 2010s: as health insurance plans and their sponsors (namely employers and government agencies) sought to reduce health care costs, they moved more financial and clinical decision-making responsibility to patients and their families, claiming that the alignment of payment and expense in the hands of the end-user of care would drive costs down.

This phenomenon was coined *consumer-driven* health care by Harvard Business School professor Regina Herzlinger, dubbed the "godmother" of the concept by *Money* magazine in 2004.[16] Herzlinger called for a consumer-based health care system back in a 1991 *Atlantic Monthly* article, "Healthy Competition," followed up by her 1997 book, *Market-Driven Health Care*.

Consumer-directed health plans were introduced in the 1990s as a backlash to highly-restrictive managed care plans, giving members more "skin in the game" in the form of greater financial exposure to health care decisions. In theory, doing so would morph patients into informed and empowered purchasers of health care based on the traditional economic theory of John Stewart Mill who conceived *Homo economicus:* rational economic man.

Patients, caregivers, and healthy people are beginning to grow consumer muscles in this transition of the U.S. health landscape. American health care is moving from a paternalistic, defined-benefit world to one of defined contribution, expressed through high-deductible health plans.

As people become more engaged health consumers, they're defining personal health across many dimensions: physical; mental, emotional, and spiritual; external appearance (how we "look" directly shapes how we feel about our health and wellbeing); and, financial. [17] The emerging health consumer isn't so much seeking to consume health care. S/he's in search of health, wellness and betterment.

Every person makes choices every day that boost, or diminish, health. Today, the health/care consumer is playing this out as they evolve into *Homo economicus* as well as *Homo informaticus*, able to tap into countless sources of information, services, and products using multiple communication channels over many platforms, increasingly digital ones.

Today, just as many people trust retailers and digital companies to help manage their personal health as they do health care providers.[18] Most people have smartphones,[19] and most people access their phone to get health care information.[20] Some 3 in 4 U.S. households have broadband connections at home,[21] and half of these people want smartphone-based medical alerts.[22] Most consumers read Nutrition Facts labels in search of healthier food,[23] and seek healthier versions of favorite foodstuffs in grocery stores.[24] To meet the demand among consumers for food-as-medicine, food retailers are hiring dietitians[25] and allocating more square footage to pharmacies, health and wellness services.[26]

In response to consumer demand, the retail health world is fast-expanding. That's happening well outside of the traditional health care system. Note that consumers made 26 trips a year to purchase over-the-counter medicines in 2015.[27] People visited doctors, on average, only three times in a year.[28] As a result, the retail store is fast becoming a logical place for health engagement.

Consumers are seeking and embracing health outside of the traditional bricks-and-mortar sites of hospitals, doctors' offices, and diagnostic centers. Health is made where people live, work, play, pray and learn: in their communities.[29] Technology is increasingly enabling care to be delivered in these more accessible, convenient, lower-cost venues that can both engage people in their own care and drive health care costs down for all payors – especially for the consumer/patient as payor.

I've written this book based on three decades of work advising organizations in the U.S. and Europe operating in every segment of the health care ecosystem: hospitals, physicians, health insurance plans, government agencies, payors, large employers, technology companies, pharmaceutical, biotechnology and medical device suppliers, financial services companies, consumer goods, food and foundations.

Over a decade ago, working on a strategic plan with one of the world's largest pharmaceutical companies, I advised that they pay closer attention to the widening copayment levels between generics and branded prescription drugs. Patient copayments for generic prescriptions were moving up from $5 to $10, and from $10 to $20 and higher for brands on health plans' approved drug lists (known as formularies). If my client's branded drug wasn't approved for inclusion on the formulary, the consumer's copay – that is, their retail out-of-pocket cost at the pharmacy cash register – would rise to $40, $50 or more, depending on the consumers' health plan type and arrangements. Surely, I suggested, this would affect consumer choice at the point-of-purchase, and the company's bottom line.

It was at that point I felt the beginnings of patients' emerging role as health consumers. I explained to the drug company senior management that the patient was transforming into a payor once that co-pay amount exceeded a twenty-dollar bill. The prescription drug began to compete, in household budgets, with other spending – like buying food, filling up a car's gas tank, paying the utility bill, or buying a birthday gift for a family member. I started my blog, *Health Populi*, at that same time in 2007 with a post featuring a sign from Tom's Shell service station with gas prices marked, "Arm," "Leg," and "First Born."

That fiscal-feeling about the spiraling cost of gas at the tank is how more American patients feel now as they morph into payors and health consumers facing growing out-of-pocket costs at the point of care -- at the pharmacy, the doctor's office, or hospital finance department. Now, patients are literally thinking about their arm, leg and first born in the larger context of household spending.

This book explains how *HealthConsuming* has come to be; how consumers are playing growing roles in making health for themselves, their families and friends, and in their communities, facing ever-growing financial health risks; peoples' growing use of mobile platforms and broadband, and the promise of digital health for self-care and health care; expanding access for retail health; the overwhelming evidence for addressing the crucial influences of the social determinants of health; growing challenges of personal health information privacy; and, ultimately, whether Americans have the prospect of becoming full health citizens like peers are in the rest of the developed world.

In America, we are all health care consumers now. Health care costs consume our bank accounts, increase our stress, disturb our sleep, decrease our wellbeing and deplete our personal and national economies. We have become aware of the burden of poor health and health expenses more than ever before and this trend is on a one-way trip, up and to the right.

What if...patients in the U.S. didn't stress over the cost of health care?
What if medical debt wasn't a key contributor to personal bankruptcy in America?

Chapter 2

THE PATIENT IS THE PAYOR

"Today's high deductibles are tomorrow's bad debt," a Moody's analyst wrote .[30]

Patients dealing with serious conditions consider cost when they look for healthcare and have postponed or avoided care due to cost. We learned this in a survey conducted among 300 activist patients in the WEGO Health community in February 2018.[31]

After we reviewed the research, we titled the study "The Empowered Patient and the Endangered Wallet" which spoke to what patients told us in the poll. The 300 people who participated in this survey were mostly female and well-educated (two-thirds had at least a Bachelor's degree and 9 percent had a PhD). These were also very experienced patients who blogged about their conditions, shared videos online with other patients, offered peers support in their patient communities, and knew how to navigate American healthcare better than most.

Half of these activist patients, all tech-savvy, sought less costly alternatives for care without their clinicians' input. Half didn't have sufficient funds available to pay for their healthcare in 2017. One-third of the patients had annual out-of-pocket costs of at least $5,000.

Of the 300 patients polled, 293 of them said the U.S. healthcare system was not sustainable as it currently functions. Most of these patients believed the U.S. should have a universal healthcare system with each individual covered by health insurance.

More worried and stressed about paying for health care than getting sick

On June 29th, 2018, a woman was injured underground at the Massachusetts Avenue subway station in Boston, blood and bone exposed through her thigh. As commuting bystanders began to phone 9-1-1, she cried out, "Do you know how much an ambulance costs?" She answered her own question: "It's $3,000. I can't afford that." A *Boston Globe* reporter witnessed the incident and wrote up the story, which was titled, "A horrific injury. A heroic rescue effort. And a desperate plea: Please don't call the ambulance, it costs too much."[32]

The reporter tweeted about the incident. That tweet garnered 9,232 retweets and 17,638 likes as this book went to press.

By 2018, Americans were more worried about the availability and affordability of health care than about crime and violence, Federal government spending, guns, drug use, hunger and homelessness, and the future of Social Security.[33] Gallup has asked this "worry" question for many years, and noted that healthcare, "is the only issue of the 11 Gallup has measured consistently to maintain this level of worry."

MORE AMERICANS ARE AFRAID OF PAYING FOR CARE THAN OF GETTING A SERIOUS ILLNESS

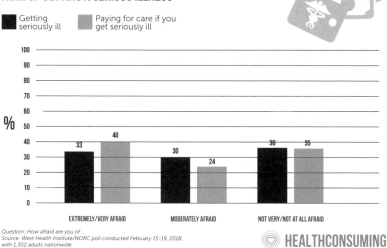

Getting seriously ill | Paying for care if you get seriously ill

	EXTREMELY/VERY AFRAID	MODERATELY AFRAID	NOT VERY/NOT AT ALL AFRAID
Getting seriously ill	33	30	36
Paying for care if you get seriously ill	40	24	35

Question: How afraid are you of ...
Source: West Health Institute/NORC poll conducted February 15-19, 2018, with 1,302 adults nationwide

HEALTHCONSUMING

For people who work and receive health insurance on the job, healthcare is also seen as the most critical issue in the United States.[34] Workers' dissatisfaction with American healthcare is based on cost, and a lack of confidence in the ability to get needed treatments, even among these Americans who received health insurance at work.

By 2018, more Americans were "extremely afraid" of paying for healthcare if they became seriously ill than of the state of becoming ill.[35]

Health care costs cause stress for most Americans, regardless of income.[36]

Consumers come to fear the prospect of incurring healthcare costs through experience with the healthcare system, as the WEGO Health patients have done. It is an American norm for people to self-ration care due to cost: to avoid going to doctor when sick, to go without routine physicals or preventive care, to skip a recommended test or treatment, or not fill a prescription for medication...all, to avoid cost.

In the growing era of consumer-directed health plans with more people enrolled in high-deductible health plans, and deductibles ratcheting upward, consumers want to know health care costs up-front.[37] Most patients say the availability of up-front cost estimates would influence their choice of a healthcare provider – the same percentage that believes bedside manner influences their choice of a doctor. The health consumer's financial experience in healthcare has gained equal weight with the patient's clinical experience with care.

In search of transparency

Transparency in the eyes of a consumer means clear communication of the direct costs for which the patient Is responsible. One in three patients told the credit bureau TransUnion they were offered a pre-treatment cost estimate, over half were confused by their medical bills, and most people were surprised by their out-of-pocket costs after-the-fact.

Forty-three of fifty U.S. states were given a grade of "F" for failing to provide a minimum standard of health care price transparency.[38] Only three states – Colorado, Maine and New Hampshire – scored "A's" for providing detailed pricing on procedures through accessible, easy-to-use public websites built on detailed data, based on the Report Card on State Price Transparency Laws sponsored by the Health Care Incentives Improvement Institute (HCI[3]) and the Catalyst for Payment Reform (CPR). The organizations emphasize that successful transparency tools are based not only on collecting data on price information, but on how states present the price information in terms of clarity and usability by consumers. The onus has been on individual state legislatures to draft and pass legislation to address health care transparency, as well as provide statewide searchable websites for healthcare prices.

Childbirth is the leading reason for hospital admissions in the U.S.,[39] and maternity is one of the most "shoppable" healthcare services. Even before becoming pregnant, a woman has time to consider her options in terms of location, reputation of the maternity program, and qualifications of the obstetricians and staff in the unit. But the costs of having a baby in a hospital can tremendously vary. Hospital costs for maternity services for low-risk pregnancies ranged from less than $2,000 to nearly $12,000 in 2015, based on an analysis of discharge data.[40]

Health care prices for maternity care vary substantially between states and within local markets; a pregnancy ultrasound researched in a study using 2015 pricing data found the national price was $268, in Alaska $895, and in Arizona, a low of $201.[41] There can also be large variations in health care prices within the same metropolitan area. The same study found that the difference between the 25th and the 75th percentiles for the ultrasound within Philadelphia was twice the difference in prices between Philadelphia ($460) and Harrisburg, PA ($234).

For maternity services, it can pay to shop around. For a consumer enrolled in a high-deductible health plan, giving birth at a high-cost hospital can significantly add to out-of-pocket costs that, with mindful comparison shopping, could be saved for other health spending. Hospitals highly value maternity patients because for many women (and their partners), the experience is the first time they have been admitted into a hospital. Thus, maternity programs in local markets often compete for patients based on high levels of service and, especially, hotel-like amenities (such as gourmet dinners with wine, spa-like environments, private birthing rooms, and interior designed tailored to the demographic). One such program launched at Miami-based Jackson Health System in 2014 and included, "quiet work spaces for dads, a coffee and tea bar with fresh pastries delivered throughout the day, and housekeeping that treats the patient like a guest on a cruise ship with towel swans."[42]

Shopping for health

Consumers know that shopping for health care is challenging, in terms of unearthing and comparing costs of different providers, predicting coverage and out-of-pocket costs, determining the best value across care options, and identifying timely discounts and savings opportunities: the very work tasks that make up "shopping."[43] But as Tina Rosenberg wrote in the New York Times, "There is practically nothing we shop for the same way we did 15 years ago. Except in healthcare. Most of us still buy blind."[44]

Shopping for an MRI may sound like a straightforward thing to do for a patient whose doctor has recommended getting that digital image to follow up a visit. But even with that very specific medical service, most patients didn't shop around for one based on price or location – they usually went to the imaging provider to whom their doctor referred them, finding that the influence of a doctor's referral is greater than the impact of a patient bearing more costs.[45]

Price shopping is possible in healthcare, other researchers found, as long as consumers receive simplified price information that is designed quite differently from typical health plan communications.[46]

Still, having high-deductible health insurance has begun to morph patients into consumers as the first-dollar payor of health care. Using what now feels like "my money," people enrolled in high-deductible health plans viscerally feel the pain of paying for health care, the way employers, government agencies, and other health insurance plan sponsors have done over the past two decades facing higher-than-general-inflation increases for health plan premiums.

But consumers still feel uncertain about making health care decisions: most people don't know how much they need to save for health care costs, and aren't confident they have maximized their health tax benefit.[47] Consumers are much more comfortable shopping for a TV, a car, picking a mobile phone provider, and booking travel themselves. Shopping for healthcare? Not so much.

When the Affordable Care Act was first implemented in 2014, uninsured consumers who could buy on health insurance exchanges for health plan coverage were also stretching new health care shopping muscles. "How bad are we at buying health insurance? Very, very bad," asked and answered a CNBC story.[48]

We live in the grand age of consumer review sites on TripAdvisor, Yelp!, and Zagat. But no such comprehensive site exists for healthcare in our local markets. Nearly 60 percent of U.S. patients believe that online reviews are important when selecting a physician.[49] A study reviewed 28 physician-rating websites in 2016, which allowed patients to leave reviews for doctors, without a subscription, enabling search by physician name.[50] The research examined a random list of 600 physicians from 3 cities – Boston, Portland, and Dallas. The study looked into 28 review sites for the sample physicians, and found a median number of 7 reviews per doctor across all sites. However, one-third of physicians had no reviews at all.

The study concluded that it is difficult for a prospective patient to find, for any given physician, a sufficient quantity of reviews that would be accurate in describing patients' experiences of care with that physician. While some engaged patients have rated doctors on Angie's List and Yelp!, among other sites, the vast majority of patients have yet to share their experiences about doctors and hospitals with other online patients.

The emergence of the patient as the payor

Most consumers view financial health as part of their overall health and wellness, along with their physical health, mental and emotional health, and personal appearance.[51] Money and finances have been among the top risk factors for for health, measured in the American Psychological Association's Stress in America Survey launched in 2007.

Stress related to financial issues has a significant impact on Americans' health and wellbeing. Financial stress and indebtedness have been shown to have negative impacts on both mental health and physical health, including heart disease, diabetes, overweight and obesity, and back pain.[52]

Most Americans have been struggling financially dealing with health care costs, according to the Center for Financial Services Innovation (CFSI).[53]

Medical bill problems can have lasting impacts on patients and families' standard of living, financial stability, and the ability to access needed health care.[54]

One-half of consumer debt in the U.S. is medical debt, the Consumer Finance Protection Bureau (CFPB) found.[55]

HEALTH CARE STRESS FELT REGARDLESS OF INCOME

No matter their household income, Americans are equally likely to say certain health-related issues are sources of stress for themselves, their loved ones or just in general.

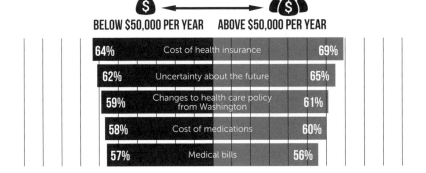

BELOW $50,000 PER YEAR   ABOVE $50,000 PER YEAR

64%	Cost of health insurance	**69%**
62%	Uncertainty about the future	**65%**
59%	Changes to health care policy from Washington	**61%**
58%	Cost of medications	**60%**
57%	Medical bills	**56%**

Note: Percentages refer to the respondents who indicated stress for themselves,
their loved ones or just in general with regard to certain health-related issues
Source: American Psychological Association

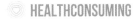

HEALTHCONSUMING

Most people having problems paying medical bills report having other kinds of debt, most commonly from credit cards, car loans, and student loans.

People enrolled in higher deductible health plans have been more likely to report medical bill problems than people with lower deductibles. Women have been more at-risk for medical bill paying challenges than men, as are younger people under 30 and adults with children in the household. Three in ten people who report medical bill problems have taken a pay cut or reported losing a job due to illnesses that led to medical problems.[56]

The CFPB found that 43 million consumers with a credit report at a national credit rating agency have at least one medical account in collection. The Bureau cautions consumers about medical debt's potential impact on FICO scores – for people with a score of 680, medical debt could reduce the score by as much as 65 points, and for those with a FICO of 780, 125 points.

Americans don't save much

The personal savings rate in the U.S. hit a high of 17.3 percent in May 1975, and a low of 2.2 percent in July 2005.[57] Since 2013, the rate has hovered between 6 and 7 percent.

The U.S. Bureau of Economic Analysis calculates the personal savings rate as the ratio of personal income saved to personal net disposable income. Let's do some simple arithmetic for further contextualizing overall personal saving with the micro-savings categories — retirement, emergency, college and healthcare. Median household income in the U.S. in November 2018 was $63,554 and the savings rate was 6%. Multiply that income by the savings rate and you get a product of $3,813.

Seven years into the economic recovery from the Great Recession, 44 percent of households told the Federal Reserve they'd have to borrow money or sell something to cover an unexpected medical cost. Four in ten people with a medical expense in that past year had debt related to cost or unpaid balances with their healthcare providers.[58]

Now, consider the following statistics on health care spending by consumers in the U.S.:

- The average annual health insurance premiums in 2018 were $6,896 for single coverage and $19,616 for family coverage.[59]
- The average annual deductible for a worker with an employer-based health plan was $4,210 for family coverage

for an employee working in a large firm and $5,862 working in a small firm in 2018.

◎ Spending per person on prescription drugs was $1,038 in 2017.[60] That's the *per capita* average based on National Health Expenditures in 2017. For context, if a patient was prescribed Gilead's Sovaldi to deal with Hepatitis C, they could be faced with paying for a single pill priced at $1,000, adding up to a total course of treatment of $84,000.[61]

The new healthcare consumer is faced with the challenge of both shopping *and* saving: shopping for the price of prescription drugs or healthcare services, and saving to pay for deductibles, out-of-pocket costs, and unanticipated medical emergencies.

Americans' relatively low savings rates, coupled with dependency on credit cards for the costs of daily living, push healthcare saving to the bottom of the household budgeting barrel. The eventual mounting of medical debt often leads to personal bankruptcy, where health care costs are a key contributor to Americans' growing financial unwellness.

The uniquely American problem of medical debt

When someone in America gets a call from a collection agency, chances are it was due to medical debt. This was the conclusion of a study from the Consumer Financial Protection Bureau which examined consumers' credit records.[62] The CFPB found that six in ten people who had been contacted by a debt collector said it was for healthcare services. Consumers who had medical debt ranged across age and income levels.[63]

Nearly one-half of U.S. families would not have $400 in an

emergency without using a credit card, borrowing from family or friends, or selling off their possessions.[64]

One of the top states for medical debt is Mississippi. A study in Mississippi found that the middle class carried more medical debt than lower income citizens.[65] The state has one of the highest percentages of adults who avoid doctor visits due to costs. Medical debt is the top cause of bankruptcy in Mississippi.

Even in Mississippi, the implementation of the Affordable Care Act had a positive impact on consumers' accumulation of medical debt. The Urban Institute found that families who had problems paying medical bills fell between 2013 and 2015, after the start of the ACA.[66]

Even with the ACA, by 2017, one-fifth of Americans still could not afford to pay an unexpected medical bill without accumulating debt.[67] Furthermore, most people have received a medical bill for which they did not budget some time in their life – more women than men, people with lower incomes, and those with less education.

The challenge of medical debt is not new – it has been a sorry feature in American healthcare for over ten years, when an analysis of the problem was published in *Health Affairs* called, "Bankruptcy Is the Tip of a Medical-Debt Iceberg."[68] This article was published in 2006, when the authors talked about medical debt being "surprisingly common." Then, medical debt was more concentrated among people who lacked health insurance.

The comedian and talk-show host John Oliver highlighted medical debt on his program, *Last Week Tonight*.[69] Oliver's team researched the medical debt buying industry, and for $50, registered a debt collection agency called Central Asset Recovery Professionals (CARP) in Mississippi in 2016. They then purchased a medical debt portfolio, worth $14.9 million, for $60,000, then gifted the portfolio to the RIP Medical Debt Charity which subsequently forgave the debt for 9,000 patients live on Oliver's show on June 5, 2016.

The hospital as collector - patients look to finance medical costs over time

The growth of high-deductible health plans, with patients paying costs out of pocket until reaching their threshold when insurance kicks in, has been a net negative for U.S. hospital finance. Hospitals have faced growing bad-debt from patients, adding staff to manage the problem. Eventually, hospitals have sold past-due accounts to collection agencies.

The patients' side of the story is that they faced a 29.4 percent increase in deductible and out-of-pocket maximum costs between 2015 and 2017. Over those two years, median wages grew 3.1 percent between 2015 to 2016, and 0.2 percent between 2016 and 2017, for a total growth of 3.3 percent compared with a nearly 30 percent increase in health care costs for patients.[70, 71] This top-line for the patient-as-payor is that healthcare costs grew about 10 times faster than wages in just the two-year period 2015 to 2017.

The process of hospitals dealing with patients' payments and receivables is known as revenue cycle management (RCM). By 2017, the challenge of bad medical debt has motivated hospitals to adopt more retail-style technology and processes to get paid.[72] "Patients truly are the new payers," noted Eric Brown of Black Book Research who conducted the research into hospitals' new approach to RCM.

Banks have spotted an opportunity to help bridge consumer medical finances with hospitals, plagued by bad debt. Some hospitals offer zero-interest loans to patients, for example. This service has been described by one healthcare trade publication as "a mortgage for healthcare costs."[73] What's driving interest among hospitals and financial service companies in this concept is the fact that the patient is now the third-largest payor in healthcare, after government and employers.

Most U.S. patients want healthcare providers to offer cost information before a procedure, and whether doctors offer financial options to help them extend payments over time.

A consumer survey from HealthFirst, a patient financing company, was titled *It's Never Too Soon to Communicate Pricing and Payment Options*. The study found that two-thirds of U.S. consumers wanted healthcare providers to discuss financing options; however, only 18 percent of providers had spoken to patients about such financial plans. At that point, only 8 percent of patients had used either zero- or low-interest financing to pay off medical bills over time.[74]

With more hospitals engaging in more retail-style payment tactics from the time a patient registers for a procedure, health economist Gerard Anderson observed, "it's an often gentler version of asking you to pay up."[75]

Crowdfunding for medical expenses

To pay out-of-pocket medical expenses, some patients have gone beyond using credit cards or borrowing from family and friends, looking to crowdfunding. Over one-third of people in the U.S. have borrowed money from friends or family to pay for health care expenses.[76] This concept is growing and scaling for healthcare through crowdfunding, as an NPR story noted in 2012.[77] Since launched in 2010, the GoFundMe site raised about $5 billion by 2016, about one-half of which was designated for healthcare.[78][79]

Crowdfunding is a method that people use to finance a project by raising money contributed by a large number of people, usually via the Internet. By 2015, 22 percent of U.S. adults had contributed money to a crowdfunding site like GoFundMe or Kickstartr.[80] Most donors to crowdfunding sites have given at most $50 to an individual project.

Crowdfunding has become a way for patients facing substantial medical bills to get financial support to pay them. Beyond medical bills, patients dealing with serious conditions can also need money for travel, rent and utilities when in the midst of combating their illnesses. By 2017, there were at least a dozen online crowdfunding sites available to patients including CauseWish, Fundly, GiveForward, GoFundMe, IndieGogo, Medgift, MyLifeLine, Rally, Thoughtful, Watsi and YourCaring.

Crowdfunding for medical expenses is a uniquely American tactic; the Financial Times explained, "American medicine is big business and the U.S. spends more on it than any other nation, yet it is the only developed country that lacks universal healthcare coverage. A fifth of U.S. household spending went on healthcare in 2013, compared with just 4 per cent in the EU, according to Eurostat, a statistics agency."[81]

The Spectrum Health's Heart & Lung Specialized Care Clinics in Grand Rapids, Michigan, directed a patient who could not afford a heart transplant procedure to use crowdfunding to pay for her surgery. The hospital's denial of coverage letter recommended that the patient organize "a fundraising effort of $10,000" to cover the high cost of immunosuppressive drugs required to prevent organ rejection.[82] Patients have been able to raise significant financial support for healthcare on these sites: GoFundMe's most successful campaign raised over $2 million through over 37,000 donations to help a patient in South Carolina with Sanfilippo syndrome, a rare neurological disease.[83]

Beyond these sites, new financial services companies are emerging to support patients in crowdfunding medical expenses. Experian launched Patient Gifting, a medical fundraising program for patients to fundraise via social networks on Facebook and Twitter. Funds raised here are funneled directly to the patients' hospitals' bank account to pay for medical expenses, thus helping the institution risk-manage bad debt due to a patient's inability to pay a bill. "It's a level of service that distinguishes your facility as being one that truly cares, not just about the episode, but the quality of patients' lives," according to the Patient Giving website.[84]

Recognizing the growth of crowdfunding for personal medical expenses, a 2017 article in *JAMA* raised ethical and legal issues about the concept.[85] Some of the authors' concerns were the potential equity divide between patients who had access to online tools and social networks versus people who lacked digital and social access. Furthermore, clinicians' lack of knowledge about crowdfunding for medical costs may beg the question of whether doctors should be responsible for supporting patients' crowdfunding efforts. Finally, there is the potential for people to engage in illicit activities, with crowdfunding's underlying emotional potency to generate sympathy and funds by providing exaggerated information, the authors warned. They pointed to a patchwork of laws which make the potential problems challenging to manage.[86]

The wage-health insurance trade-off

Employer-sponsored health insurance covers over one-half of working-age Americans.[87] Leading up to the 2016 Presidential election, whether one identified as a Democrat or Republican, Americans' paychecks had stayed relatively flat for well over a decade. At the same time, healthcare costs grew very quickly. Over those years, workers essentially traded off wage increases so they could receive health benefits at work as part of their total compensation package.[88] This turned out to be an implicit, if not transparent, social contract between workers and employers from the late 1990s through the Great Recession and its aftermath.

The cost of coinsurance for healthcare services and supplies like prescription drugs increased by 107 percent over the ten years, 2004 to 2014. Wages increased only 32 percent over that decade.[89] And it wasn't as if benefits got richer; in fact, health benefits got less generous, with narrowing provider networks, slimmer prescription drug formularies, and limits on various medical services and supplies.

The trade-off between personal wage stagnation versus hockey-stick growth of health care costs translated into a financial risk-shift from companies to workers.

A new car, college, or health insurance?

The shrinking American middle class saw their health care costs increase while spending on other household line items fell. Peoples' spending on all basic needs such as clothing, food, housing and transportation dropped as healthcare costs were rising.[90]

People used many strategies to pay for health care in 2015.[91] The

FOR OVER A DECADE, WORKING AMERICANS HAVE TRADED OFF WAGE INCREASES FOR HEALTH INSURANCE COVERAGE

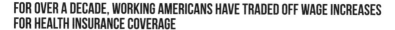

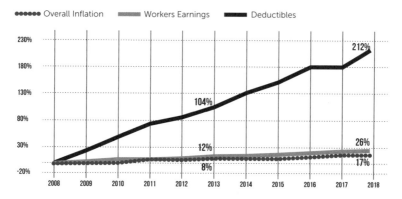

Note: Average general annual deductibles are among all covered workers. Workers in plans without a general annual deductible for in-network services are assigned a value of zero.

Source: KFF and KFF/HRET Employer Health Benefits Surveys. Consumer Price Index, U.S. City Average of Annual Inflation (April to April); Seasonally Adjusted Data from the Current Employment Statistics Survey (April to April)

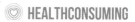

most common tactic to pay for medical bills was to put off vacations or other major household purchases, like washing machines and automobiles, along with cutting back spending on food, clothing, and basic household items. Over one-half of people drained savings to pay for health care in 2015. One-third of people took on extra hours at work or a second job.

But there was another pretty desperate strategy that one-fourth of people used to pay medical bills: they withdrew money from retirement, college, or other long-term savings accounts. That is, simply put, raiding savings *for future benefit* (in retirement, for children's college education, or for emergency use) to pay *for current health spending.*

Most surprising about this tactic: while 1 in 4 of all consumers took money out of retirement to pay for healthcare, doing this was more common among people who had health insurance – one in three of whom withdrew money from a 401(k) or college savings plan. Financial planners refer to this as a "401(k) medical hardship."

When it comes to savings behavior, consumers are more focused on putting money away in retirement accounts and emergency funds, followed by saving for kids' college. This reveals consumers' savings preference for items other than healthcare. The bottom-line on savings in America: 50 percent of consumers made contributions toward retirement each month, two times the number of people that saved for healthcare.[92]

Around 2010, there began to be an obvious financial risk-shift from business to consumers as a response to companies bearing larger healthcare cost increases charged by insurance companies to sponsor employee health plans. While double-digit price increases for health insurance have since dropped into the single-digits, the cost for covering a family of four through a preferred provider organization plan design hit $28,166 in 2018.[93] With that money, an auto buyer could purchase a new Subaru Crosstrek SUV, pay for a year of college at Texas Tech University, or put cash into a down payment on a home.

Self-rationing due to cost: fiscal vs. physical

The costs of medical care have compelled people in America to take steps that self-ration, avoiding or postponing some aspect of medical care. While it's understandable that people without health insurance might delay or avoid getting healthcare services, self-rationing also happens among people with insurance who have trouble paying medical bills.[94]

More than half of Americans delayed medical care between 2017 and 2018 because they couldn't afford it. Nearly half of consumers also admitted their health takes a back seat to other financial obligations.[95] While it's more common for people with lower incomes to avoid healthcare due to cost, some 16 percent of consumers earning over $100,000 a year did so, too.

Most people in a Bankrate survey admitted to living paycheck to paycheck.[96]

The medical irony of postponing necessary health care due to current costs, whether splitting pills to conserve them for future use or avoiding getting a recommended medical test, is that in the cause of rational short-term *fiscal* avoidance, longer-term adverse *physical* consequences can result which would cost the consumer-patient even more money and time downstream.

Self-rationing health care due to cost is a serious challenge for people managing chronic conditions, for whom postponing or opting out of care due to cost can lead to longer-term medical complications and even higher health care costs. Financial barriers negatively impact heart disease patients' ability to self-manage cardiovascular disease, contributing to patients' non-adherence to medicines and self-care.[97] Patients who perceive a financial barrier for health care also had higher rates of hospitalizations and higher hospital costs than patients without perceived financial barriers.[98]

Gallup's research found that two-thirds of people who put off medical treatment in 2017 were dealing with serious conditions. More women than men delayed medical treatment due to cost, as well.[99]

The high costs of prescription drugs: a toxic side effect

Some 45 million Americans did not fill a prescription in 2016 due to the cost of medications.[100] This rate of prescription drug self-rationing is nine times greater than that in the United Kingdom, where the National Health Service covers most of the costs of prescription drugs.

Consumer Reports learned that patients whose drug prices rose in the last year experienced reduced quality of life compared with people whose drug costs did not increase. Those impacts had to do with having less disposable income to spend on entertainment and dining out, buying groceries, spending less on families, postponing bills, and using a credit card more often.[101]

Doctors working at Memorial Sloan-Kettering Medical Center called out "financial toxicity" as an observed side-effect of cancer. In health care, financial toxicity is the impact of a disease or medical treatment on a patient's net worth and debt. The concept of financial toxicity for cancer patients was raised by concerned clinicians at the Medical Center, who discussed the topic on the CBS News program *60 Minutes* in 2014.[102]

The National Cancer Institute found that one in three patients with cancer has turned to family or friends to help pay for their medical care, putting families at-risk for financial hardship. Between 33 and 80 percent of cancer survivors exhaust savings to finance medical expenses.[103] atients surviving colon cancer in Washington State had an average level of debt of $26,860.[104] Bankruptcy among cancer survivors was 2.5 times greater than among households without a cancer patient.[105] Furthermore, financial toxicity also adversely impacts the risk of dying: cancer patients who filed for bankruptcy had a 79 percent greater mortality rate versus people with the same diagnosis who did not go bankrupt.[106]

Beyond strong medicines, the new financial toxicity in America is also due to the impact of the cost of hospital inpatient admissions on household budgets. The rate of bankruptcies in the U.S. increased in the years after hospital admission, both one and four years after the admission.[107] A team of researchers from academic medical centers underscored this financial wellness challenge in a 2018 peer-reviewed paper titled, "Death or Debt? National Estimates of Financial Toxicity in Persons with Newly-Diagnosed Cancer."[108] The study estimated that about 9.5 million newly-diagnosed people with cancer over 50 years of age were impacted by financial toxicity.

The sting of EpiPen prices: the birth of the healthcare consumer

A story published on the "Passages" page of *People* magazine dated September 12, 2016, took me by surprise. That's the part of the magazine featuring stories about celebrities' births, deaths, divorces, and marriages; the Circle of Life stuff. But this paragraph made me stop in my reading tracks: *"HEALTH: EpiPen manufacturer Mylan raised the price of the allergy injector to more than $500 – a 400 percent increase since they started selling the product in 2007. Public outrage ensued. The company then announced that it will soon start selling a generic version of the product for half the price."*

This, in *People* magazine with a cover story about Rob Kardashian.[109] Then, I saw a satire in *MAD* magazine about EpiPen pricing called, "Reasons Why the Price of EpiPens Increased." The first reason given was that, "Extensive market research showed that people are willing to pay a little more to make sure that they don't suffocate and die."[110]

I knew as I re-read about the EpiPen in pop culture magazines that my many years of forecasting emerging health care consumerism had reached a tipping point.

The mainstream driving force underneath that story was the fact that the EpiPen price increased from $94 in 2007 to $608 in 2016. This product is purchased by millions of moms and dads in America every year to ensure their kids' allergies to peanuts and bee stings don't have fatal consequences. Parents took to blogs, parenting forums and online chats to channel their rage. One Mom interviewed on NPR called the EpiPen price hike "a matter of life and death."[111] Eventually, EpiPen buyers crowdsourced that rage into market power.

Months later, Mylan, the drug's manufacturer, introduced a generic EpiPen priced at $300. "We cut the price in half," company CEO Heather Bresch (daughter of U.S. Senator of West Virginia, Joe Manchin) told CNBC, "We took action with the EpiPen. It's half the price."[112]

CVS/health, the pharmacy chain, reduced the cost by offering a rival generic version: they dropped the price to $109.99 for a two-pack, one-sixth of the original price.[113]

By February 2017, generic competitors to the EpiPen hit the market and together took market share away from Mylan: in December 2016, 5.3 percent of epinephrine auto-injector prescriptions went to alternatives for EpiPen. This nearly tripled in January 2017, and hit close to 30 percent by the end of February 2017.[114]

The lesson: don't mess with EpiPen-buying parents, fiercely fighting for their kids' health and access to medicines. Increasingly, the healthcare industry will be confronting patients and caregivers who, faced with more direct out-of-pocket costs, will be growing health consumer and political activist muscles.

In the meantime, Margot Sanger-Katz offered this advice in her

New York Times column: "Here is the surest way to enjoy the peace of mind that comes with having health insurance: Don't get sick."[115]

*What if ... healthcare looked and felt
more like an Amazon experience?*

Chapter 3

HOW AMAZON HAS PRIMED HEALTH CONSUMERS

Healthcare doesn't feel like Amazon

In 2016, consumers told Aflac that enrolling in health insurance should feel like an experience on Amazon.[116] But healthcare experiences, whether shopping for and enrolling in health insurance, dealing with pharmacies, or sorting out hospital bills, just don't feel like Amazon to American patients.

Consider the organizations that garnered the most consumer brand loyalty in 2018: of the top ten, nine were technology companies. The tenth, Trader Joe's, is all about food, value and fun.[117]

The heads-up for the healthcare industry is that every one of these brands does something related or adjacent to health — perhaps with the exception of Netflix, unless you consider movie-watching therapeutic (which my household definitely does). Each of the top brand companies is also rewiring the consumer experience for better service in retail, daily living, communicating, and...health.

ONE-HALF OF AMERICANS THINK BUYING HEALTH CARE SHOULD FEEL LIKE AN AMAZON EXPERIENCE

In an ideal world, my benefits enrollment process would be more like ...

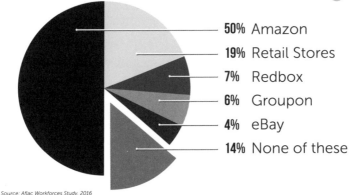

- **50%** Amazon
- **19%** Retail Stores
- **7%** Redbox
- **6%** Groupon
- **4%** eBay
- **14%** None of these

Source: Aflac Workforces Study, 2016

Respondents chose from: Amazon.com, with easy-to-compare options online; A retail store, where I can talk to someone and make my purchase in person; Redbox, with a variety of options available at a kiosk where I shop; Groupon, with daily deals; eBay, with auction pricing; and none of these.

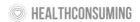 HEALTHCONSUMING

In 2018, the Temkin Experience Ratings found high scores for supermarket chains, fast food, retail, banks, parcel delivery, streaming media and hotels. The lowest experience ratings went to TV and internet service providers, and health insurance plans.[118] The Temkin index is based on how a consumer rates an organization on success (how well an experience meets customer needs), effort (how easy it is for a customer to do what she wants to do), and emotion (how does the customer feel about the experience).

Put that lens over the healthcare experience:

- Do organizations serving health consumers meet their needs?
- Do healthcare organizations make it easy for health consumers to do what they want/need to do?
- How do health consumers feel about their experiences with healthcare in America?

One simple metric gives you a sense of healthcare's lack of delight: wait times for appointments. In 2017, patients seeking a new doctor's appointment waited an average of 24 days to get it scheduled.[119] Boston wait times were longest, at 52 days; Dallas wait times for doctor's appointments were the shortest at about 15 days. Other average wait times were 37 days in Philadelphia, 28 in Portland, 28 in Seattle, 27 in Denver and 24 in Los Angeles. In smaller, mid-sized cities, wait times averaged 32 days, one-third longer than in major metropolitan areas.

That's nothing like an Amazon Prime experience, which has set a high new-normal bar for customer service.

We are all *Homo informaticus* now

TIME magazine crowned "You" as the Person of the Year in 2006.[120] The subtext was that, by going online, searching the World Wide Web, You, the people, controlled the information age. Lev Grossman wrote, "It's a story about community and collaboration on a scale never seen before. It's about the cosmic compendium of knowledge Wikipedia and the million-channel people's network YouTube and the online metropolis MySpace. It's about the many wresting power from the few and helping one another for nothing and how that will not only change the world, but also change the way the world changes."

By 2017, the average American home had five Internet-connected devices.[121] Three in five of these devices were smartphones; other connected technologies included computers (desktop or laptop), tablets, and streaming media devices (like Amazon Fire TV, Apple TV, or Roku).

Peoples' use of the Internet, coupled with the fast-adoption of smartphones, have morphed us from *Homo sapiens* into *Homo informaticus*.[122] Most people manage aspects of everyday life using several technology platforms.

We are information omnivores, going omnichannel in daily life at work, for entertainment, to shop, to learn. People expect this omnichannel experience in healthcare, too.

How Amazon has primed health consumers

Consumers are Amazon-primed now. So it should not surprise healthcare providers, plans and suppliers that consumers expect just-in-time convenience for their healthcare. "Consumers are clear: In the 21st century, 20th century healthcare is not good enough," where technology can enable the modern patient to choose when and how they receive health care services, an Accenture consumer survey learned.[123]

Mind this gap: the demand side is clearly in favor of more healthcare delivered virtually, digitally, more quickly, and less costly. On the supply side, though, there's been a lag in providing virtual care, notwithstanding consumers' collective wish for technology-enabled services.

Amazon Prime members now outnumber non-Prime accounts. Over one-half of U.S. households were subscribed to Amazon Prime in 2019.[124] Globally, there were 100 million Prime members, Jeff Bezos, Founder and CEO, wrote in a letter to shareholders.[125] The number of Prime subscribers could more than double to 275 million by 2028, Citi forecasted.[126] Prime members spent on average $1,300 a year on about 25 purchases, compared with non-Prime shoppers who spent $700 on 14 occasions.[127]

Members know that they can receive an item labelled "Prime" in the marketplace within two days of ordering it (if not sooner), what their total charges will be for that item before checking out, and what other consumers who have purchased the item think about it based on customer reviews posted on the site.

That Amazon experience has raised peoples' expectations for goods and services they pay for outside of the Amazon store... including healthcare. "The last great shopping experience drives a customer's expectation for the next," Steve Laughlin, General Manager, IBM Global Consumer Industries, has observed.[128]

It's natural that the EveryMan and EveryWoman, now all part of the species *Homo informaticus,* would ask, "why can't accessing healthcare services and my personal health information be as easy as dealing with Amazon?"

The Amazon priming of consumers is animating their demand for more accessible, quality-vetted, and transparently priced healthcare.

Alexa and voice-tech: from digital assistant to health assistant

Voice-enabled digital assistants are emerging as Internet of Things hardware that can support people's health-making at home.

Amazon's voice-enabled personal assistants dominated the U.S. market in 2018, accounting for about seven in every ten devices [129] (competing with Google Assistant, Microsoft Cortana, Apple Siri and Samsung Bixby). Note that while Prime membership bolsters Amazon shopping to the tune of $1,300 on average per member per year, owning an Amazon assistant raises that annual spend to

$1,700.[130] (This fact may be why these devices are often priced as loss-leaders to promote their consumer purchase and adoption).

By early 2018, 39 million people in the U.S. owned a voice-enabled digital assistant, separate from a voice assistant on their smartphone. Digital assistants help consumers manage all sorts of personal tasks: calling up recipes, playing music, offering directions, updating weather and answering the questions, "Alexa, what time should I take my next pill" and "Alexa, how can I eat fewer carbs at breakfast today?"

Half of those adopting voice assistants in 2017 used them for some aspect of their health care: to ask about symptoms they were experiencing, to access diet tips, to connect to a health care provider, or to inquire into health insurance options, among many health-voice interactions.[131]

Introduced in June 2015 to Amazon Prime subscribers, the Amazon Echo found early adoption for health applications. "Alexa's best skill could be as a home health-care assistant," a CNBC analyst reported, finding that home health aides using the digital assistant could help clients better manage medications and support family caregivers.[132] The Libertana Alexa skill was developed by Orbita, a voice platform company founded by two software developers each of whom had aging parents with complex health challenges.

Digital virtual assistants like Alexa, Cortana, Google Assistant, and Siri are especially popular among young parents.[133] BabyCenter polled parents on the role of voice-controlled and Internet of Things devices, learning that the majority of parents owned at least one such device in early 2017, and many felt they were better parents due to the electronic devices. Why? Connected devices made their lives easier, saved time, and gave parents more control. One major motivation was for the devices to help people save money.

To that end, one of Amazon Alexa's skills was developed to help people locate cheaper prescription drugs. By calling on Alexa to summon GoodRx, the consumer (patient) speaks a prescription drug name and the GoodRx app, via Alexa's voice, identifies common doses of the drug, where the drug can be purchased at the lowest price in the community, and provides the range of costs at nearby pharmacies. For example, a search for Crestor conducted in December 2017 found a price range between $14.45 and $225.64, with generic statins at the low-end.[134]

Providers have also been working with Alexa on how digital assistants can help make healthcare better and cheaper.[135] Hospitals throughout the U.S. have been testing out these devices with patients. "If you are an inpatient, what are the things typically you would like to know?" queried John Halamka, MD, Chief Information Officer at BIDMC. "When will my doctor be here? What's for lunch?" he posed. "Alexa? Ask BIDMC what is my diet?" And Alexa replies, "You are restricted to a bland diet for the day. To order a meal, call extension 12345."

Northwell Health developed an Alexa skill to help people assess wait times for the emergency room. Commonwealth Care Alliance created an application running over Alexa that helps patients access their inpatient schedules for the day. Libertana Home Health worked on voice-tools to help patients age independently at home.

Alexa is but one connection in a growing ecosystem of devices that are forming the Internet of Healthy Things at home, further discussed in the *Digital Health* chapter.

Health as a growth strategy for Amazon

Health consumers are hungry for Amazon's brand of transparency, convenience, and streamlined interactions for medical care. The Amazon Prime-ing of the U.S. consumer has raised peoples' expectations of what health care services *could* be: personalized, customized, anticipatory, immediate or on-schedule, and convenient – where we live, work, play, pray, learn and even drive.

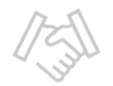

MORE CONSUMERS ARE GROWING COMFORTABLE WITH AMAZON AS A HEALTH CARE SUPPLIER FOR PRODUCTS, SERVICES, AND MEDICINES

Consumer trust levels for Amazon

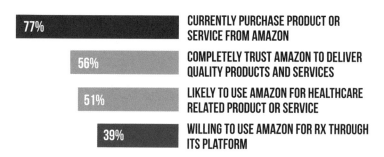

77%	CURRENTLY PURCHASE PRODUCT OR SERVICE FROM AMAZON
56%	COMPLETELY TRUST AMAZON TO DELIVER QUALITY PRODUCTS AND SERVICES
51%	LIKELY TO USE AMAZON FOR HEALTHCARE RELATED PRODUCT OR SERVICE
39%	WILLING TO USE AMAZON FOR RX THROUGH ITS PLATFORM

Source: Market Strategies, Amazon Is At It Again: Disrupting Healthcare and Pharma, July 2018

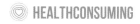 **HEALTHCONSUMING**

While Amazon has set that new customer experience bar for healthcare consumers, the company is also expanding its portfolio of projects in the health/care ecosystem beyond voice. Amazon first made a foray into the legacy healthcare system in 2000 when the company invested in Drugstore.com to enter the pharmacy business.[136] Drugstore.com was the first internet retailer on Amazon which received bullish headlines supporting the venture like, "Farewell, Preparation H aisle.[137] But the timing for that ambition was too early, and the venture was dissolved in 2005.[138]

Many years later, Amazon seems to think the timing is right to expand their healthcare efforts. At the start of 2019, the company was disrupting the traditional healthcare landscape across industry stakeholders by:

- Expanding the over-the-counter medicines business, Basic Care, competing with retail pharmacy, Big Box, and grocery stores
- Distributing medical supplies to doctors and hospitals, competing with the largest publicly traded healthcare distribution companies (including the ability for a customer to use a DASH button for automatic fulfillment or using Alexa to shop by voice)
- Going direct-to-consumers to sell medical supplies to chronically ill patients through the Xealth platform
- Advancing work on electronic health records through Comprehend Medical, which analyzes patients' EHR data
- Evolving Alexa tools for medical and wellness applications; in 2018, Amazon filed a patent for Alexa to analyze users' speech and emotions, and recommend treatments to consumers who may sound unwell[139]
- Allying with JPMorgan Chase and Berkshire Hathaway with Dr. Atul Gawande at the helm of a project to lower healthcare costs and improve experience for employers and workers receiving health insurance through the workplace
- Extending AWS web services to healthcare organizations looking to store data in the cloud
- Reimagining the pharmacy benefits business (PBMs)
- Expanding the company's Solimo label of nutritional supplements and personal care items through the Elements private label brand [140]
- Leveraging its investment in PillPack, the prescription drug delivery service

- Offering discounts for Prime membership to people enrolled in Medicaid or SNAP benefits (a tactic that could help address the challenge of food deserts in areas lacking access to nutritious groceries).

These projects illustrate the growing nature of health@retail, which Amazon will play a role in both defining and serving. But Amazon is also inspiring and challenging health care incumbents as well as new entrants to build new business models and services that meet, anticipate, and exceed consumers' expectations for wellness and medicine.

The Amazon effect may have motivated vertical integrations and mergers, such as the CVS + Aetna and CIGNA + Express Scripts deals. In addition, Best Buy's acquisition of GreatCall re-defines the retailer's blur from channeling products to providing services. Walgreens' partnership with FedEx for fast-delivery of medicines, Walmart allying with Philips and T-Mobile for telehealth, and Lyft and Uber serving as transporters for health care providers are other examples repositioning health care for higher levels of consumer service. Bedfellows that may seem "strange" in today's health care ecosystem aren't so out-of-place in a consumer-centered health and wellness world.

What if ... healthcare happened where we live, work, play, pray and shop, delivering the highest levels of retail experience?

Chapter 4

THE NEW RETAIL HEALTH

Barbershops, places of worship, and grocery stores: the new front doors to health

Once upon a time, the barbershop pole outside a storefront on Main Street was a sign that you could enter the shop and receive healthcare – from healing a cut to getting a compound cream for a skin condition, along with a haircut.

Some barbershops have begun to revive that tradition. One shop in Wilmington, North Carolina, Just Cut It, has collaborated with the New Hanover Regional Medical to provide flu shots and blood pressure screenings.[141] Barbers working in a St. Louis barbershop-for-health program became "true believers" in preventive care, learning that the black barbershop was a trusted source of health information.[142]

Why is this *déjà vu* healthcare strategy so powerful? Because, "the barbershop has always been such a social staple in our

HEALTH IS EVERYWHERE - COMMUNITIES HAVE MANY TOUCHPOINTS FOR HEALTH BEYOND HEALTHCARE

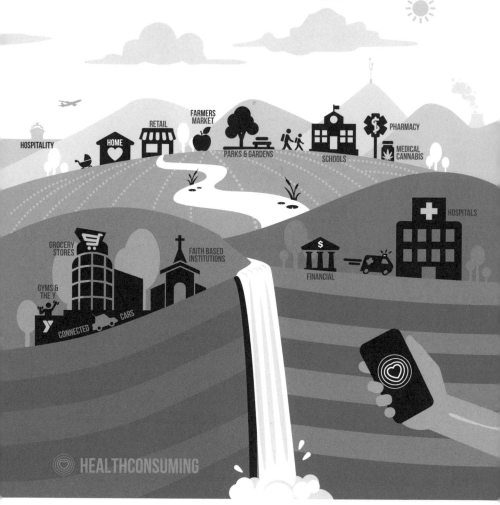

community," according to Jermaine Armour, a client of Just Cut It who took advantage of getting healthcare at the barbershop.

"It's refreshing to get outside those hospital walls," Joshua Jones, a pharmacist who works at the barbershop with clients, observed. "This is more in peoples' home environment, so they are more relaxed."

Jones knows that people would rather not be so-called "health consumers", but just people going about their way, day-to-day, living life on their own terms outside of the medical system. This is true whether people seek primary care, like flu shots or sore throat remedies, or to access mental health services in a non-taboo environment.

Enter the Frazzled Café in the United Kingdom, where people meet to exchange personal stories and share stresses. Marks & Spencer, the British retailer, hosts Frazzled Café meet-ups around the UK.[143] Frazzled Café's tagline is, "It's OK not to be OK," and Marks & Spencer extends stores' café spaces as places where people can feel that sharing is safe.

"Retail" as a direct-to-consumer health concept can also include faith-based institutions, which have long played roles as front-doors to health – both spiritual and physical.[144] The role of faith has been studied as a social determinant of health among public health professionals.[145] Beyond religiously-branded hospitals and care facilities, faith-based organizations provide chaplaincy and spiritual outreach to parishioners and residents, congregational health promotion and disease prevention, and food security in their communities. The National Academy of Sciences, Engineering and Medicine convened a workshop in 2018 to learn about faith's role in improving population health, assessing how "scientific wisdom" could couple with "faith wisdom" to improve health outcomes in communities.[146]

Retail spaces, community centers and public places are becoming the new front doors to health, as more patients seek self-care options that are more convenient, accessible, price-transparent, engaging, reflective of personal values – and value.

The post-Recession consumer: more self-reliant

National health spending in the U.S. hit $3.7 trillion in 2018, with money going to hospitals, doctors, prescription drugs, long-term care, and other services that get paid for through insurance company health care claims, government programs like Medicare, Medicaid and the VA, and consumers' share of premiums, copayments, and coinsurance payments.

But consumers spend more than what's in the health insurance claim. U.S. patients-as-consumers spent additional funds on *health,* on stuff like vitamins and supplements, fitness club memberships, chiropractors, massage therapists, weight loss programs, wearable technologies and other goods and services to bolster wellness. Little of this spending was reimbursed by health insurance.

The Great Recession of 2008 shook the financial ground beneath the American economy. Once U.S. consumers found their sea-legs after these economic tremors, people were fundamentally reshaped. Nearly 3 in 4 Americans either lost a job or had a relative or close friend who did since the advent of the financial downturn.[147]

According to research published in the aptly titled study, *Eyes Wide Open, Wallet Half Shut,*[148] the post-recession consumer sought greater value, creativity, sustainability, and health.

A do-it-yourself ethos blurred into peoples' approach to health: the Great Recession drove people to increase online health searches, especially for chest, headache, heart, pain, and stomach issues. There were 200 million more online health queries during the recession, according to researchers who analyzed web searches for health topics among post-recession consumers.[149] Searches for stomach ulcer symptoms and headache symptoms were over two-times greater than would have been expected.

The bottom-line: after the Great Recession hit, Ogilvy observed, "self-reliance is the new insurance policy."[150]

Consumers' self-reliant streak, when coupled with well-designed digital self-service programs, can lead to higher levels of consumer satisfaction. People have become so digitally self-reliant that most would rather use a company website than make a phone call or send an email for customer service.[151] In fact, a majority of consumers would rather solve their own problems online than rely on a company's live call center.[152]

We feel like Rodney Dangerfield when it comes to our healthcare

People feel like get-no-respect Rodney Dangerfield when they deal with health insurance, government agencies, and pharma companies. Consumers feel much more love from personal care and beauty companies, grocery and fitness centers, according to C Space's study into what people value in a brand.[153]

Nine of the top 10 companies that C Space identified with the highest customer value were adjacent in some way to health: grocers (Publix, Wegmans, Trader Joe's, H-E-B), personal care and beauty companies (Dove, Olay), hospitality/travel (Marriott), fitness (REI), and one healthcare organization: St. Jude. The next ten organizations featured more personal care, travel, fitness along with financial services (which, when done right, can bolster financial wellness).

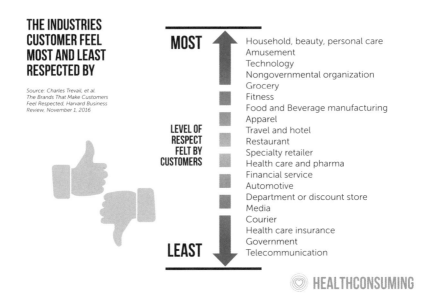

THE INDUSTRIES CUSTOMER FEEL MOST AND LEAST RESPECTED BY

Source: Charles Trevail, et al.
The Brands That Make Customers
Feel Respected, Harvard Business
Review, November 1, 2016

MOST

LEVEL OF RESPECT FELT BY CUSTOMERS

LEAST

Household, beauty, personal care
Amusement
Technology
Nongovernmental organization
Grocery
Fitness
Food and Beverage manufacturing
Apparel
Travel and hotel
Restaurant
Specialty retailer
Health care and pharma
Financial service
Automotive
Department or discount store
Media
Courier
Health care insurance
Government
Telecommunication

HEALTHCONSUMING

Consumers seek health engagement everywhere

On average, a person in the U.S. sees a doctor three times a year.[154] For people over 65, it's seven doctor's appointments annually. For people 25 to 44 years of age, it's twice a year. If you're a baby under one-year old, you see the doctor on average over seven times a year.

That means through about 360 days of the year, we're not in a doctor's office. So health is created largely outside of the health care system: health is where we live, work, play, and pray.[155]

Consumers intuitively get that. We look for health beyond hospitals, doctors' offices, and medicines. People want to engage for their health across the full range of industries: with food and beverage manufacturers, media and entertainment, consumer electronics, retail, and even brewing and spirits companies and financial services.[156] This extends to peoples' expectation that all kinds of companies should engage in health beyond helping their own employees with health insurance and wellness programs.

When it comes to placing trust in companies to help people manage their health, equal numbers of consumers polled trusted large retailers, digital companies, and healthcare providers.[157] The reasons why are key lessons for the traditional legacy healthcare industry: transparency in quality and price (preferably, low) and a clear, understandable value proposition. Consumers understand what they are going to get when they click into a search box on an ecommerce site, type in a desired commodity, and receive a list of options showing a clear picture of the item, price, description, and consumer ratings. That shopping process and experience communicates transparency of price and explains the benefits of the product. In healthcare, such a dashboard has been missing in action. While several companies have received hundreds of millions of dollars of venture funding to build such a capability, these tools haven't yet yielded the rich dataset, functionality and usability that people need to be true health consumers.

The growth of retail health "front doors"

There's a growing list of new front doors, in Oliver Wyman's words, for people to enter for healthcare that are designed with peoples' retail expectations in mind. People see these sites as more convenient, cheaper, price-transparent, and digitally-enabled.[158]

The traditional doors to primary and urgent care have been the doctor's office, hospital ambulatory clinics, and the emergency room. Today, that front door to care can be:

◎   An urgent care or retail medicine clinic, in a pharmacy, at school, in a hotel or overseas tourism destination;

- Virtual, via telehealth, video-visits with doctors, nurses, or health coaches (akin to Skyping with a clinician), or at a health kiosk; or,
- At home, receiving a new kind of medical house call, along with other creative entrances (bricks and virtual) for health services.

So the new front door for healthcare isn't really a physical door: it's, optimally, a well-designed, touchpoint for health directly accessed by the consumer. Most consumers who have used these retail health alternatives usually like them: eight in ten people who used either urgent care or a retail clinic said they received about the same or better care experience as in a traditional healthcare setting. And as people take cash out of their wallet to pay for health services and products, they're seeking retail-style experiences with the bar set by their favorite ecommerce sites like Amazon, grocers like Publix and Wegmans, and banks like Regions (Temkin's top-rated bank for customer experience).

Retail clinics

The most expensive front door for healthcare is the emergency room. Now that patients are payors, there has been a substantial shift among patients moving from the high-cost ER to lower-cost acute care alternatives: to retail clinics, urgent care centers, and telemedicine options.[159] Retail clinics are not only less expensive per visit, but deliver primary care in convenient places. At least one-quarter of emergency department visits could take place at an urgent care center or retail clinic.[160]

About 2,000 retail clinics operated in the U.S. in 2018.[161] These providers are usually located in drugstores, supermarkets, and big box stores. Retail clinics' typical business has been treating low-acuity conditions: upper respiratory issues, ear infections, urinary tract infections, dermatology, and conjunctivitis, among other complaints. These clinics have also become a significant provider of vaccinations and immunizations. Retail clinics are typically staffed by nurse practitioners, registered nurses who have advanced training and, depending on the state they work in, can prescribe drugs.

Retail clinics deliver at least as high a caliber of care as doctor's offices do, according to studies by Ateev Mehrotra of the Harvard Medical School. Dr. Mehrotra has found that retail clinics often follow clinical practice guidelines more faithfully than physicians do.[162] Furthermore, patient experience can be more highly rated in retail clinics than in doctors' offices, due to convenience and the fact that the clinic staff can take more time with patients, driving experience scores higher.[163]

Clinics are especially popular with parents of young children because pediatricians' offices are generally closed in the evenings and weekends – when children's symptoms for common infections often flare (think: high fever at 11 pm on a weeknight, or on a Sunday morning). As the author of a *New York Times* opinion column with young children at home wrote about such a situation, "My wife and I both work...If physicians want to reclaim that business, they will probably have to offer the same benefits of scheduling and efficiency that retail clinics do."[164]

Retail clinic services are going well beyond screening for infections and completing school health forms. Some major chains operating retail clinics have developed clinical affiliations with academic medical centers and hospital systems in local markets, and are providing more chronic care management and services dealing with lifestyle behavior changes such as smoking cessation support and obesity management.[165]

Urgent care centers

There were more than 8,100 urgent care centers operating in the U.S. in 2017.[166] Urgent care centers are typically physician-staffed, and treat more acute illnesses and injuries than retail clinics. Urgent care fills a role between primary care and the hospital emergency room. The Urgent Care Association of America (UCAOA) has developed criteria for credentialing urgent care centers, which include accepting walk-in patients, being open 7 days a week, being staffed by a licensed physician, treating a broad spectrum of illnesses and injuries, having on-site diagnostic equipment (e.g., X-ray), among other features.[167]

Urgent care centers can be owned by hospitals and health systems as well as other healthcare companies; by local physicians and entrepreneurs; and, by urgent care companies that operate chains of centers regionally or nationally. Dignity Health, a health system operating in Arizona, California, and Nevada, acquired the urgent care company U.S. Healthworks to extend its delivery networks into patients' communities. HCA and Tenet, two for-profit hospital companies, also entered the urgent care market. UnitedHealth Group's Optum division began to develop urgent care centers under the brand name MedExpress in Minnesota in 2016.[168]

Traditional health care providers have noticed their patients' growing use of retail and urgent care clinics. As a result, health systems have acquired these sites or have struck alliances with them to keep patients within their clinical "family" which helps to retain those patients in the hospitals' healthcare systems.[169]

As retail clinics and urgent care centers mature and provide services complementing hospitals, they are using more sophisticated electronic health record (EHR) systems.[170] Exchange data between urgent care and hospitals will become increasingly important as centers assume a bigger role in patients' healthcare continuity.

The Doctors Office 2.0 - new clinic models

The primary care appointment is being reinvented by a new kind of clinic model that at first looks more like a living room than your doctor's waiting room. One Medical, "Sherpaa Health (which Crossover Health acquired in February 2019), CareMore Health, and Iora Health, among others, take a customer service page out of Zappos' playbook rather than one from the typical physician's office.

"One Medical has an industry-leading 91 Net Promoter Score (NPS) and retains over 88 percent of its consumer members and 99 percent of its enterprise employer partnerships," a recent press release announced about the company's round of $350 million funding.[171]

There aren't many healthcare organizations who talk about Net Promoter Scores as part of their business and investor strategy this way.

While each of these new-fangled clinic organizations has their unique branding, they have been designed and built with technology, convenience and efficiency from their inception. The new clinic models tend to be underpinned by electronic records, internally developed based on the practice's workflow and team-based care processes. Patients book appointments online, pay automatically with a credit or debit card, and have access to their personal health information online.

There are new-style practices being expressly developed for women, too, getting a makeover in both brick-and-mortar offices and virtual clinics. Tia, a direct-pay membership model, launched in New York City in 2019 as an "in-network" provider for OB-GYN and primary care accepting major insurance plans. In addition to the usual medical services on offer, Tia Clinic members also have access to a mobile health record, acupuncture, meditation and stress management, and kombucha on tap. That's targeted marketing.

Maven is a virtual clinic with a downloadable app which is freely downloadable and free to use. Maven hosts a directory of over 1,200 women's and family practitioners across 18 specialties. The user can select a provider, and meet them virtually via smartphone or computer. As of late 2018, visit prices ranged $35 for a ten-minute chat with a doctor, $50 for a 30-minute appointment with a baby sleep coach, and $70 for a 40-minute meet-up with a therapist.

Health at the pharmacy

Over 90 percent of people in the U.S. live within 5 miles of a pharmacy.[172] This is a major reason the pharmacy can be relevant and accessible to support people in making health close to home, work, and play.

There are over 67,000 pharmacy storefronts in America, and mostly all of them go well beyond dispensaries for prescription drugs.[173] One-third of pharmacies are chain drugstores, and another third are independent pharmacies. The remaining third of retail pharmacies are located in supermarkets and mass merchant stores.[174] Many retail pharmacies and their operators were listed on the Fortune list of largest companies in America in 2018 including Walmart (#1), CVS Health (#7), Costco (#15), Kroger (#17), Walgreens (#19), Target (#39), Publix (#88), Rite Aid (#94), Weis Markets (#668), and Fred's Super Dollar (#942).[175]

Pharmacies benefit from a key leverage point other retail health touchpoints don't have: the pharmacist. That profession is among the highest-rated for ethics across all other job categories; except for nurses, pharmacists have been among the top-ranked professions for honesty and ethics in America since the Gallup Poll posed the question.[176]

Pharmacies can build on their trusted pharmacist-consumer relationship as accessible storefronts for health, wellness, and healthcare: they've been called "the face of neighborhood healthcare."[177] Pharmacies are growing the core mission of dispensing medications to build end-to-end healthcare services that help people move across the continuum from prevention to sick care.

Take medication adherence. Adherence is the extent to which a patient follows recommendations for prescribed treatments. Non-adherence to prescription drug instructions costs nearly $300 billion a year in the U.S. and contributes to some of the 125,000 deaths due to unintended adverse events.[178] That $300 billion approaches nearly 10 percent of total U.S. health care spending.

Pharmacies have become popular sites for immunizations. Most Americans over the age of 35 would prefer getting a shot at a community pharmacy than from a doctor's office.[179] It's all about convenience: and that's what's driving so much innovation at your neighborhood drugstore: a pharmacy can be a one-stop shop for health and wellness, it's usually easier to get to than a doctor's office, and service tends to be faster and more friendly in a retail environment.

To ensure continuity of care between hospital and home, pharmacies are also partnering with medical systems and health plans. Community pharmacists interact with consumers more than healthcare providers do and are in a good position to help patients coordinate healthcare in daily life, like the barbershop Just Cut It mentioned at the start of this chapter.

While current U.S. federal law does not recognize pharmacists as healthcare providers, the American Pharmacists Association is advocating for legislation that allows pharmacists to provide care in under-served communities. Four states (California, Montana, New Mexico and North Carolina) have expanded pharmacists' responsibilities to include providing primary care.[180]

The drugstore is also growing as an ecommerce touchpoint beyond Main Street and strip malls, as digital drugstores expand bricks-and-mortar access online. The largest pharmacy chains, along with Amazon, are expanding online capabilities for filling, re-filling, and distributing prescription drugs.[181]

2018 was the year of a big shift for retail pharmacy. Amazon's 2018 acquisition of PillPack for $1 billion enabled the company to launch its footprint in digital pharmacy across the U.S.[182]

To ensure they continue to play a role beyond bricks-and-mortar pharmacy, CVS Health and Walgreens, the two largest chains in the U.S., expanded well beyond their legacy pharmacy businesses. CVS Health merged with Aetna, the health insurer, vertically integrating many components of health care services. Walgreens launched several new initiatives, including offering telehealth on demand, collaborating with Kroger on a new concept grocery store combining pharmacy and food in a smaller footprint, partnering with Humana, the health plan, and expanding its beauty segment by working with Birchbox.

And, to compete with Amazon and PillPack, both companies began to offer next-day or faster home delivery for prescription drugs to patients' homes in 2018.

Historically, the retail pharmacy chains have achieved high levels of customer satisfaction, J.D. Power has found.[183] "U.S. consumers love their pharmacies," J.D. Power noted. Consumer satisfaction scores for pharmacies rank with the highest scoring industries. One of the most impactful drivers of customer satisfaction in the pharmacy was "non-pharmacist staff greeting you in a friendly manner," J.D. Power identified.

Hospital-ity: a growing market for healthy hotels and wellness travel

Retail health extends beyond medical care locations like doctors' offices, hospitals and clinics. People who travel, for both business and leisure-pleasure, are looking for wellness baked into destinations well outside of traditional healthcare sites. One-third of travelers are motivated to pursue wellness programs and healthy lifestyles.[184]

Several drivers underlie the growing interest in wellness travel: high among these factors is peoples' feeling of stress and burn-out whether from work, finances, social, or political sources.

Wellness travelers are coping by seeking out opportunities to slow down. The rising popularity of yoga and wellness retreats are part of a growing business of helping customers unplug from the Internet and the always-on lifestyle.[185]

The wellness tourism market grew at 14 percent between 2017 and 2018, twice as quickly as the overall tourism sector.[186]

Wellness travel is defined as vacationing while enhancing or maintaining one's well-being, whether physical, mental, or spiritual, according to the Global Wellness Institute. Traditionally, spa resorts have been the obvious wellness travel product, but the category is expanding from beauty and restfulness to active fitness classes, yoga and meditation, personalized nutrition offered at Canyon Ranch's locations, and the WellnessFX program at Cal-a-Vie which analyzes a client's blood to assess cardiovascular, hormonal, metabolic and nutritional health.[187]

The hospitality industry, which includes hotels, airlines, cruising and restaurants, sees health and wellness as a growth lever. To meet consumer demand for health, the hospitality sector looks to address good sleep through curating beds, in-room exercise options, healthy food on restaurant menus, and outdoor areas for yoga.[48] Wellness travelers' expectations go way beyond the 85 percent of hotels that have a fitness center equipped with a few stationary cycles, treadmills and free weights.[189]

"Having the pool guy teach yoga just won't fly anymore," one report on the renaissance of hotel fitness options observed. [190]

All of the major hotel brands have created wellness concepts, and not just because doing so might have a positive halo effect on their business. Wellness travelers have been found to be willing to spend a premium over average rack rates — at least $20 a night more for a wellness-designed hotel room.[191]

Some examples illustrate hotel chains' varied approaches to serve wellness travelers. InterContinental Hotels Group launched the EVEN Hotels brand for wellness. Hotel employees host small group exercise classes, and guest rooms come with a "fitness zone" outfitted with a yoga mat, strength-training bands, exercise ball and fitness videos.[192] To enter wellness with a mature brand, Hyatt acquired the Miraval Group, a pioneer in wellness hospitality through its spa resorts in Tucson (the Miraval Arizona Resort) and Austin (the Travaasa Resort), for $215 million, in 2017.[193] Hyatt also created a new position for a senior vice president, global head of well-being, to address both guest and employee wellness.[194]

AccorHotels re-defined its luxury concept with wellness in mind. Various of the chain's properties offer healthy cooking classes, "super-foods" on restaurant menus, full moon yoga, and a Vitality Room in Swissôtels in collaboration with *Wallpaper* magazine. Westin collaborated with New Balance, the athletic wear company, to provide workout gear (including sneakers) to lodgers at various properties. The Soho House and W Hotel in Los Angeles, and The Great Northern hotel in London, allied with Barry's Bootcamp, a California-based workout company. SoulCycle, the cardio-boosting indoor cycling studio, works with hotels across North America.[195]

Wellness in the hospitality industry is going beyond hotels. While better-known for midnight buffets that may bust healthy diet goals, cruise ships have expanded wellness offerings at-sea. Cruise lines have typically offered spa services as a major revenue stream on-board. But there's a new-and-improved menu of wellness and healthcare on cruise ships these days.

Canyon Ranch, the well-known spa brand, boarded the Regent Seven

Seas Explorer in 2016 bringing its SpaClub at Sea to wellness-oriented cruise passengers. Some of the wellness opportunities available on a Mediterranean Cruise include a Tai Chi class in the Imperial Garden of the Pharo Palace in Marseiiles, France; yoga and meditation around Mount Etna in Taormina, Sicily; hydrothermal therapy in Civitavecchia, Rome, soaking in mineral-rich springs visited by Kings and Popes over one thousand years; and aromatherapy in Amalfi, spending time at the Carthusia perfume lab.[196]

The Seabourn line has collaborated with Dr. Andrew Weil and his integrative medicine approach on ships that sail Alaska and the Mediterranean. Seabourn brands these experiences as Wellness Cruises with Dr. Andrew Weil, and brings integrative medicine colleagues into mindful living programs at sea including a Mindful Living coach. In October 2018, Dr. Weil led a cruise on the Origins of Wellness around the Mediterranean.[197]

In 2019, the first wellness cruise line, Blue World Voyages, set sail, remaking a 900-passenger cruise ship into one housing 350 clients with one of the highest spa-to-passenger ratios in the industry. The ship features high-def golf and soccer simulators, studios for yoga, spinning and TRX, battling cages, along with other fitness activities. On-land excursions specialized in active trips and the ability to anchor at smaller remote harbors due to the relatively small footprint of the ship. Healthy cuisine was developed with chefs from Chez Panisse, Charlie Trotter's, and Tra Vigne (from Napa Valley).[198]

From sea to the air, airlines and airports are also marketing to wellness travelers via healthier food options, sleep amenities, and relaxation opportunities. Delta Air Lines offers the Deepak Chopra Dream Weaver guided meditation program at the Asanda Spa Lounge in Sky Clubs at JFK airport in New York and the Seattle-

Tacoma Airport. Quantus provides an in-air meditation program to help passengers relax on long air hauls. Singapore Airlines partners with Canyon Ranch for healthy food in the skies. At least ten airports offered spaces for yoga in 2018. Be Relax, Roam Fitness, and Yoga on the Fly ("your ticket to traveling well") host fitness storefronts in airports.

Gyms, Health Clubs, and the Y

Consumers value gyms and health clubs for supporting personal health and wellness goals: over 70 million U.S. consumers belonged to a health club in 2017. That was one in five Americans ages 6 and older, using their clubs an average of 100 days a year.[199]

Fitness conscious Americans exercise at least twice a week, and most would work out even if they felt fit and healthy without the exercise.[200] Three in four physically active Americans work out to improve their mental state and to relieve stress, and most intend to teach fitness as a priority to children. Over half of fitness-active people say prioritizing fitness is a requirement in a potential partner.

Public policy and behavioral economics can also be used to nudge people toward healthy behaviors like being more physically active. The 115th Congress House of Representatives passed the Personal Health Investment Today Act (PHIT Act) in July 2018 which allowed people with Health Savings Accounts to write off up to $500 a year for gym memberships and fitness classes as part of their medical expense deduction along with fees for youth camps, sports leagues, and marathon/triathlon registration fees.[201] The legislation had bipartisan support, sponsored by Senators Chris Murphy (D-CT) and John Thune (R-SD), and Congressmen Ron Kind (D-WI) and Jason Smith (R-MO).

Two-thirds of people who belong to a health club are members of a national chain, including a YMCA/YWCA. Members of "Y's" are the most loyal, with the lowest levels of churn (drop-out or intention to) across the various types of gyms.[202]

Research has shown that health club membership can be associated with improving cardiovascular health and physical activity.[203] A study analyzed health club members with respect to heart health measures including resting blood pressure, resting heart rate, body mass index, waist circumference, and cardiorespiratory fitness. Belonging to a health club led to significantly increased aerobic and resistance physical activity levels and more favorable cardiovascular health outcomes compared to non-members. People with a health club membership were significantly more active and less sedentary.

The Y brands itself nationally as a community-based organization committed to improving communities' health. The Y offers a broad range of health-and-wellness programs available at one of the 2,700 Y's located in over 10,000 communities. For example, the YMCA collaborates with the American Heart Association (AHA) and the American Medical Association (AMA) on a blood pressure self-monitoring program called Target:BP, led by Y-trained Healthy Heart Ambassadors who demonstrate how to use a blood pressure monitor, support self-monitoring, and conduct monthly nutrition education meetings.[204] The program is part of a broader Y initiative to bring science-based programs to under-served communities.

The YMCA launched the Diabetes Prevention Program (DPP) in 2012. The Y's DPP is a 12-month evidence-based program that has grown a national footprint. The program received a Health Care Innovation Award from the Centers for Medicare and Medicaid Services to provide the DPP to Medicare enrollees with prediabetes in participating YMCA networks. The program was found to save $278 per participating member per quarter, decreasing inpatient hospital admissions and emergency department visits.[205]

Y's are intimately woven into their local communities, with the ability to integrate and co-locate programs that can support public health. An ambitious plan for the YMCA of Greater Louisville is such an example as a community health hub. The plan is the culmination of nearly a decade of visioning and $28 million worth of financing for a new 62,000 square foot building sited in west Louisville at the corner of Broadway and 18th Streets. The project will also add about one-half million dollars' worth of salaries to the local economy and job tally. "Our vision is to create community-integrated health through the lens of health equity, in alignment with the Y's overall mission," Steve Tarver, president & CEO of the YMCA of Greater Louisville, said.[206] The Y is building a broad definition of health through partners: Norton Healthcare (hospital system), Republic Bank & Trust, Family & Children's Place (mental health services), ProRehab Physical Therapy, and the University of Louisville. Note that Altria/Phillip Morris USA originally donated the land, where a tobacco plant once stood for 50 years. "We don't just want to be a place for people to go get services; we want to be a place for youth development, for healthy living, and for other socially responsible things to take place," Tarver envisioned.[207]

Medical cannabis at retail

A 2018 Quinnipiac University poll found that 93 percent of Americans supported doctor-prescribed marijuana use.[208] Thirty-three U.S. states and the District of Columbia had legalized medical marijuana by 2018.[209] The U.S. market for medical cannabis is expected to grow over 13 percent a year from 2018 to 2024, when the value is projected to be worth $8 billion. Three quarters of medicinal marijuana was prescribed for pain management in 2017.[210] In the era of opioid addiction, associated with lethal side effects, the growing prevalence of chronic pain associated with arthritis, cancer, HIV/AIDS, and neurological disorders are drivers of demand in the U.S. medical marijuana market. Four in ten people who use cannabis do so for medical reasons.[211]

Baby Boomers are a growing customer base for medical cannabis. Aging boomers dealing more with pain get familiar with available pain-killers and inflammatory options in the "traditional pharmacopeia," and are looking for healthier, natural alternatives.[212]

Medical cannabis users will come to the experience seeking a variety of effects, from anxiety relief and treatment of chronic pain to prevention of epileptic seizures.[213]

In the context of Baby Boomers and aging America, note that medical marijuana laws may have been a factor in reducing Medicare Part D costs in states that have legalized medical cannabis.[214]

Medical marijuana is generally distributed to consumers through dispensaries. In the U.S., cannabis dispensaries are regulated by state governments. They tend to be located in convenient retail or office locations. Patients visit these shops to fill a prescription for a cannabis dose based on their physician's recommendation.

In 2019, MedMen was the largest company operating in medical cannabis in the U.S., with a strong retail brand throughout the country. MedMen is licensed for 66 retail stores across 12 states that cover 50 percent of the U.S. population. The company's dispensaries have been characterized as the Apple Stores of the cannabis industry with a high-service retail store experience.[215]

The nascent industry is building customer service benchmarks like other retailers. Cannvas Medtech developed a platform called Cannvas.me to enable users to access medical cannabis education materials and share personal data on experiences. Lift & Co.'s platform is positioned as a kind of TripAdvisor for cannabis; the site aggregates consumer reviews, shares content, and informs decisions. The company is developing a Netflix-like tool using artificial intelligence to offer consumers product suggestions.[216]

Cannabis is, in the words of JWT, "undergoing a massive rebrand, shedding its stoner image to become part of a chic, wellness-forward lifestyle."[217] To that objective, the pot tourism business is growing in places like California and Colorado, as well as Canada. In 2016, some 15 percent (13.5 million) of Colorado's 90 million visitors participated in a pot tourism activity.[218]

Shopping malls

Healthcare is reinvigorating real estate, based on a trend in shopping and strip malls repurposing for medical and wellness services.[219] Credit Suisse forecasted that up to 25 percent of U.S. shopping malls would close by 2022, signaling a potential "mallpocalypse" to real estate analysts.[220]

Health care services have begun to move into malls across America, such as the Dana-Farber Cancer Institute leasing one-half of the former Atrium Mall in Chestnut Hill, Massachusetts, and the Southeastern Regional Medical Center moving into the Biggs Park Mall in Lumberton, NC.

When fully operational in 2019, Dana-Farber at the Life Time Center will provide clinical trials and services for newly-diagnosed cancer patients. "It's a great opportunity for collaboration and to think about cancer care and wellness together," Wendy

Gettleman, Dana-Farber's vice president for facilities management and real estate, told the *Boston Globe*, noting the proximity to the fitness center as an added amenity for patients.[221]

SRMC spent $5.6 million in 2011 to expand its services at Biggs Park Mall, in a space that once occupied a Winn-Dixie grocery store. SRMC developed a health mall concept including a walk-in clinic, weight loss center, a lab, a pharmacy, community health services and diabetes education, and a surgical center. Note that SRMC also operates walk-in clinics at the town's Walmart and the Lumberton Drug store.[222]

Why would providers like Dana-Farber and Southeastern Regional site healthcare services in vacant shopping mall space? It's the convenience and access that real estate options offer. JLL, a real estate advisor, recommends that health care organizations adopt a patient-centered real estate strategy: that is, to put convenience on center stage to increase patient accessibility, recognizing that hospitals are learning from retailers by making it easier for patients to "stop in" for care. The migration of care continues to flow from inpatient to outpatient care, with a greater scrutiny on siting services that are accessible, convenient, and designed with patient experience and brand loyalty in mind.[223]

There's also tangible value that healthcare brings to mall developers and owners: not only do healthcare organizations in shopping centers bring in patients who can patronize the mall's commercial tenants, but so can doctors, nurses, allied professionals, support staff as consumers outside of the workplace.

The mall is becoming more than a new location for a medical office building. Healthcare providers are siting a broad range of services at malls, such as emergency rooms, labs, imaging centers, community outreach, and micro-hospitals.

Gyms are also finding malls to be valuable locations for consumers who want to couple exercise with retail and dining opportunities. The gym has the opportunity to channel health services to local communities. Malls have begun to court gyms to fill empty anchor store space.[224] There's evidence that people who work out are more likely to shop afterward because it has become socially acceptable to wear fitness clothing outside a gym (known as "athleisure" apparel, a market served by Athleta, Lululemon, and Fabletics, among other brands).

The Westfield group operates 33 malls in the US: over half of them have a health club onsite. The Westfield UTC mall in San Diego hosts a SoulCycle studio located by two restaurants that service organic and locally-source foods. "We're thinking of this as an ecosystem," Westfield's head of leasing noted. "It's not just a workout."[225]

The grocery store as health destination

Another form of real estate is also getting the gym treatment: grocery stores. Orangetheory collaborated with Hy-Vee, a Midwestern U.S. grocery chain, to build workout studios co-located with neighborhood stores.[226]

The Edelman Health Engagement Barometer found that nine in ten people look to the food industry to engage on health. Just as many consumers look to engage for health with food and beverage companies as they do pharmaceutical manufacturers, healthcare providers, and personal care companies.[227]

Consumers' use of food and beverages for self-care follows

closely behind healthcare and personal care consumption, and well above exercise, sleep, and natural/organic remedies.[228] Sixty percent of consumers believe that food is just as powerful as medicine when it comes to healing and treating illness.

Consumers are looking to food purchases that can prevent and/or manage disease states. Some people focus on heart health, buying up garlic, broccoli, asparagus, and kale. Other consumers want to prevent or better control diabetes, picking more citrus fruits and beans. Some consumers have increased intake of turmeric and flax seeds to combat cancer.[229] Increasing protein to deliver positive nutrition benefits is also a growing consumer health strategy at retail, where research into seafood has brought more shoppers to the grocer's fish counter.

While taste ranks the top purchase driver for food shopping, price and health tie for second-place. The price issue is central to consumers' perceptions about their ability to afford healthy food. One-half of Americans have purchased less healthy food than they would otherwise do because they don't have enough money to buy healthier food options. Nearly 1 in 2 people have also delayed grocery shopping due to other expenses in their household like utility bills and rent, or purchased less food overall because they didn't have enough money in their budget.

As a direct result of medical or prescription expenses, one-third of Americans have delayed buying food or purchased less food.

"We are trying to get to a place where food can bring medicine-like qualities," Mike Lee of The Future Market told the 2018 Partnership for a Healthier America Summit.[230] "There is an aspiration that companies are grasping at [for] food to be the answer, not medicine."

Most people diagnosed with at least one chronic condition also have an "appetite for health." Over two-thirds of older adults are dealing with at least one condition, looking to nutrition to help manage their illnesses.[231] What's exciting to hear among older people is that the vast majority believe it's "never too late" to make diet and lifestyle changes.[232] The key health benefits consumers seek from food are cardiovascular health, weight management, energy, brain function, diabetes management, and digestive health.[233]

The food-as-medicine trend has grown as patients-as-consumers seek to complement or, if possible, substitute, food and eating styles for prescription drugs when diagnosed with a condition that may be amenable to a lifestyle change, first and foremost diet. Taking a page out of Hippocrates, "let food be thy medicine and medicine be thy food," consumers are increasingly shopping for groceries with an appetite for health.[234]

The opportunity for grocers as health destinations is that, "Grocery shopping remains the all-American pastime," David Fikes of the Center for Food Integrity has said.[235] Grocery shoppers look to food stores to support their wellness, as people define "eating well" in terms of health, taste and social connection.[236] As a result, people look to food retailers to support their goals of eating well, notably in two ways: to make products more affordable, and to provide healthier choices.

What's behind these multi-pronged retail health-and-food strategies is the realization that, "to eat well, one must first shop well."[237] Many grocers have expanded their shelf space to accommodate consumers' health and wellness goals (and willingness to spend). Walmart, pioneer of the $4 generic prescription back in 2006, is leveraging its large scale for health and wellness. Each week, about 140 million shoppers in the U.S. coming through Walmart stores' doors and Walmart.com. The company's health and wellness footprint is broad, from the pharmacy to health and beauty aisles, durable medical equipment and clinics offering primary care and urgent care. Walmart hosts "Wellness Days" offering free screening and consultations for blood pressure, body mass index, diabetes and immunizations. Walmart opened a supercenter store footprint in southern Cook County, Illinois, in 2016 — a USDA designated food desert, also adding 340 local jobs with the store opening.[238] Walmart has mental health services and telehealth in its sights, as well.

Kroger has assembled a wellness offering through store pharmacists, registered dietitians, nurse practitioners and physician assistants. The grocer's Wellness Your Way platform is a website featuring healthy recipes, links to The Little Clinic (Kroger's retail clinic brand), and information about pharmacy services and over-the-counter products. The OptUP app enables the user to scan foods in the store and guide consumers to make healthier food choices, as well as track progress over time. The president of the pharmacy referred to this tool as a, "balanced, holistic approach to self-care."[239]

Kroger's pharmacy has also collaborated with the healthcare system linking store pharmacists with community physicians' EHRs. Bringing the grocery store pharmacist data beyond the prescription — such as a patient's lab tests and information about co-morbidities — improved both workflow efficiencies and patient outcomes.[240] Further growing its position in the healthcare ecosystem, Kroger developed the Rx Savings Club, a pharmacy membership discount program for consumers to use when their out-of-pocket copayment might be more expensive than the discounted price for the drug at the grocery store.[241] Working in partnership with GoodRx, the program was based on the fact that for Medicare enrollees, it can be cheaper to pay a discounted cash price for a drug than acquire the product through their Part D Medicare plan.[242]

Aldi, the German-based grocer that entered the U.S. in Iowa in 1976, is the eighth largest retailer in the world.[243] Aldi expanded its health-conscious product line in 2018 which was considered the biggest refresh in the chain's history since its founding in 1954. Aldi expanded options for organic, vegan and vegetarian lifestyles. CNN reported, "Aldi (is) going granola to compete with Whole Foods."[244] The company enlarged its health-oriented food portfolio, including private labels Earth Grown (vegan and vegetarian line), SimplyNature (organic foods), Never Any! antibiotic-, hormone- and steroid-free meats, and liveGfree (gluten-free foods).

Coborn's, a grocer operating in the upper Midwest, offers complimentary consultations for shoppers managing diabetes, high blood pressure, allergies, among other health issues. They offer shoppers a healthy check-out lane which features wellness products and no high-sugar or salty snacks. The company's weight management program serves both employees and shoppers, with the aim of informing and inspiring healthy changes in eating patterns, positive feelings about body image, and ultimately, reduced health care costs.[245]

Hy-Vee opened its first HealthMarket in West Des Moines, Iowa, in 2018, stocking the grocery store aisles with healthy food items along with health amenities: a pharmacy, a retail clinic, a hearing aid center, and a 3,000-square food Orangetheory Fitness center with a sports nutrition area. The HealthMarket also features a hydration station with nitro coffee, kombucha and Bevi-infused waters. Hy-Vee plans to grow this concept in its other geographic markets in the eight Midwestern states where the grocer operates, expanding first to Kansas City and Madison, Wisconsin.[246]

H-E-B operates about 400 stores in Texas and Mexico, and has a strong focus on wellness. The grocer offers wellness group classes, health education sessions, and grocery shopping tours led by registered dietitians or nutritionists who guide consumers to strategically navigate the store and learn to read food nutrition labels. For consumers who cannot or don't want to receive education at a bricks-and-mortar store, H-E-B offers telehealth appointments with store dietitians for virtual consultations. Topics cover food allergies, athletic performance, family and child nutrition, weight management, diabetes management, and digestive health.

Increasingly, grocers and other retail health touch points are going beyond bricks-and-mortar to meet consumers' omnichannel demands -- via digital health.

What if...digital health tools could scale needed health care services and reach the people who need them?

Chapter 5

DIGITAL HEALTH - WEARABLE, SHAREABLE, VIRTUAL

Learning about e-Patients from Dr. Tom

In 2007, Dr. Tom Ferguson published the first paper about the growing phenomenon of people empowered by health information titled, *e-Patients: how they can help us heal health care.*[247]

He started writing about patient-powered healthcare in 1975 and became the section editor of health, medicine and self-care for the *Whole Earth Catalog*. "DocTom" advocated that people engage in well-informed self-care, encouraging physicians to partner with patients. He had a vision of the patient as a net-savvy, well-connected, doctor-collaborative end-user.[248] DocTom sadly passed away too soon in 2006 to witness the mainstreaming of that connected health consumer.

Mainstream health consumers are evolving into e-Patients, where the 'e' can mean: equipped, enabled, empowered, engaged, equal (in the medical team with clinicians and other medical professionals), emancipated, expert, economic, and evaluating. That health engagement is enabled through digital technology, and especially mobile-first.

Going digital for self-health is as common for moms on Main Street as Millennials in Manhattan. Most Americans are active digital health adopters, using mobile health apps, telemedicine, and wearable technology.[249] Over one-half of Americans who searched online for information about their symptoms have then proposed their own diagnosis to their physician based on that information. This phenomenon has acquired its own name: "paging Doctor Google."[250]

Most people sought information online about prescription drugs, diagnoses, supplements and treatment options in 2016. Half of people acted upon this information, Rock Health found.[251] Before asking a healthcare provider, most people also looked to the Internet when they had a health-related question in 2017. Increasingly, that search was mobile: 85 percent of those who searched health information online used a smartphone or tablet to find that answer.[252]

People consider consumer electronics to be the most innovative industry they know. But people also believe that the healthcare industry should be the most innovative sector in the economy.[253]

Consumer and provider-sponsored listservs and internet community patient groups gained traction in the 1990s, heralding an era where seeking health information online has become a normal task of being a patient: eight in ten internet-connected U.S. adults used some form of digital health technology in 2016.[254]

Most consumers now use mobile phones as their platform of choice for digital media, turning less to desktop and laptop computers. By 2017, mobile accounted for two-thirds of all digital media time spent, equal to two hours and 51 minutes spent via mobile.

Nearly every consumer owns a smartphone, and by 2017, most people began to cut cords to landlines in favor of having just one phone number: a mobile one.[255] Smartphones behave like powerful computers in our pockets, pocketbooks, and backpacks because they are in fact more robust and multi-tasking than the desktops and laptops sold a decade ago. They also go where people go.

On their mobile devices, consumers arrange travel for airlines and hotels via transportation and hospitality portals as well as Airbnb; manage personal finances on Mint.com, banking and investment firm portals; organize and develop photos online; and, book restaurant reservations via OpenTable. The fastest-growing apps in 2017 were services that sought to improve existing daily life-flows, like getting directions (Waze), hailing taxis (Uber and Lyft), paying friends (Venmo), and shopping (via Flipp, OfferUp, and Wish).[256]

The same patients, consumers and caregivers who lead digital lives outside of healthcare are increasingly demanding that their healthcare experiences feel like the other parts of their lives.   By 2018, there were about 318,000 healthcare mobile apps available in app stores that smartphone users could download.[257]

Going mobile for health – patients as *Phono sapiens*[258]

"As I see it, people don't adopt mobile devices; they *marry* them," B.J. Fogg wrote in his manifesto on persuasive technology. An expert on behavior change (and how difficult it is), Fogg has studied the benefits of texting for health and using technology to persuade people to adopt and sustain healthy behaviors.[259] There is a growing body of evidence supporting the use of mobile phone apps for health, nutrition (to increase sustained changes in diet), wellness and lifestyle behavior change (to quit smoking), mental health (to reduce anxiety or stress), and perioperative care (following cardiac surgery).[260]

The opportunity to go mobile for health is that most consumers have smartphones that can connect to the Internet, and most people keep their phones within arm's reach, 24x7, in always-on connectivity.[261] The average mobile phone user looked at their mobile device at least 150 times a day, equal to every six minutes during a waking day of 16 hours.[262]

"Smartphones are the wellness delivery channel of the future," Dr. John Mattison, the Chief Medical Information Officer of Kaiser-Permanente, has said.[263] He is right, since over half of U.S. consumers use mobile platforms (smartphones or tablets) to manage some aspect of their health and this number keeps rising.[264]

How might a smartphone support an everyday person engage in their self-care to drive a personal health outcome? Consider the truck drivers who have downloaded and used the mobile app Healthy Trucker. Healthy Trucker was developed by NAL Insurance of Canada in response to high medical claims filed by professional truckers. The program poses health challenges to drivers such as eating well at truck stops, exercising on the road, and managing stress. This social network baked into self-tracking has added a motivational element beyond simply tracking that boosts engagement and continued use of the tool, resulting in weight loss, better medical metrics like improved blood pressure and cholesterol, and emotional wellness.[265]

Most people want to use their smartphones to interact with healthcare providers.[266] Some of the growth in consumers' use of mobile health apps is due to physicians recommending (or "prescribing") their patients' use of the tools to track a health or fitness metric: one in five physicians did so in 2015.

Mobile phone apps can help people track personal health metrics that are generated by wearables, diagnostic technologies, and remote health monitors. Caffeine intake, flights of stairs, heart rate, hydration, medications, menstrual cycle, mindfulness, mood, sexual activity, sleep quality and symptoms are among a long list of items not typically captured in the doctor's office or hospital clinic.

But smartphones and apps can do more than track activity and clinical data about us: these devices, backed with algorithms, can infer aspects of our health status based on that data, and provide useful guidance to inform care decisions.

Phones are, "a very good proxy for capturing how we interact with our environment and other people," observed Dr. John Torous, co-director of the digital psychiatry program at Beth Israel Deaconess Medical Center in Boston. In studying peoples' use of their phones, Dr. Torous has found that simple changes in our daily routines – from how far we travel in a day to how we're sleeping – can reveal early warning signs of mental and physical health problems.[267]

With 150 phone check-in points every day, furthered by passive sensor inputs that can add rich health context, consumers have a powerful tool for health engagement in their pocket. Patients may see their doctors three times a year for about fifteen minutes, on average, in the U.S. That's why digital health expert Dr. Eric Topol of Scripps Health has said, "We mainly rely on getting data from people coming into a doctor's office, and that's one of the most contrived environments you can imagine."[268]

Patients managing multiple conditions, like the chronic trifecta of diabetes, high blood pressure, and depression, can receive text message reminders for medication management to help coordinate complex drug-taking regimens throughout each day and potentially mitigate the risk of adverse events. Athletes training for performance can track miles run, nutrition, and hydration to prepare for their next race via their smartphone, coupled with an Apple Watch armed with mobile health apps like MapMyRun, My Fitness Pal, and iHydrate.

The digital experience is so pervasive that we have reached a point where giving up one's smartphone could actually be bad for your health. Researchers point out that smartphones allow people to improve health by accessing information and tools that can help us manage our health and, potentially, save money while doing it.[269]

One of the key reasons the mobile phone can serve as a wellness channel is that most people keep their device no more than an arm's length away during waking hours. 91 percent of people keep their mobile phones at arm's length 24x7.[270] With consumers age 55 and over the fastest-growing population adopting mobile phones, there's an expanding opportunity to support peoples' healthy aging and chronic disease management, a need which increases as people age.

Dr. Joseph Kvedar of the Center for Connected Health, has observed this in his research into virtual health care:[271] "The future of patient engagement in healthcare will be mobile. We're going to see this whole idea of engagement get more and more tied to mobile health and mobile devices....If I can get my health message in your path while you're working on your mobile device, I have a much better likelihood of engaging with you, as long as that message is personal, as long as it's relevant, as long as it helps you do something that you want to do to improve your life."

Digital, virtual health can boost access to healthcare services and enable self-care

Digital technology is on the cusp of profoundly changing how we utilize health care services and make health for ourselves and our loved ones.

The shortage and maldistribution of primary care in America puts the digital health opportunity into practical perspective. The U.S. will be short between 40,800 and 104,900 physicians by 2030.[272] This phenomenon is particularly acute in more rural communities. The shortage of primary care and other medical specialists will worsen as the population ages and grows. While the Association of American Medical Colleges, which projects the physician shortfall, believes that training more doctors is a key part of the solution, consumers' adoption and use of digital health tools, including remote monitoring and telehealth, will be crucial to expanding access to health care services and enabling self-care – which can help drive better health outcomes and experiences, and reduce costs.

Self-care is an important linchpin for realizing the full promise of virtual health care. Without patients — people, consumers, caregivers all — taking on some responsibility and action on behalf of our own health, the U.S. won't be able to lower the rate of health care cost increases.

"Well-informed patients can help lift the burden of care from the shoulders of overworked clinicians," Dr. Tom wrote. "They can do their own lab tests. They can examine their kids' sore ears with a home otoscope, listen to their own hearts to monitor an arrhythmia, administer their own peritoneal dialysis, give themselves injections, and can safely choose and self-administer many drugs currently available only by prescription."[273]

The annual CES features the latest models of cars, televisions, and home appliances (the annual trade show of the Consumer Technology Association). Since 2010, among the fastest-growing product lines unveiled at the world's largest consumer electronics meet-up have been digital health tools.[274] Activity monitors, led by Fitbit, and biosensors that read blood pressure, temperature, blood glucose, weight, and heart function, are exhibited alongside smart refrigerators and connected cars. And even the refrigerators and cars had health-related aspects to them.

CES 2019: KEY CATEGORIES IN CONSUMER-FACING HEALTH DEVICES AND THE GROWTH OF THE INTERNET OF THINGS IN HEALTH/CARE

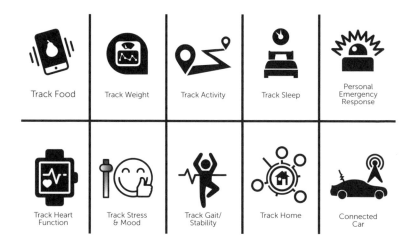

| Track Food | Track Weight | Track Activity | Track Sleep | Personal Emergency Response |
| Track Heart Function | Track Stress & Mood | Track Gait/ Stability | Track Home | Connected Car |

Source: Jane Sarasohn-Kahn, THINK-Health, February 2019

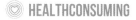 HEALTHCONSUMING

The Food and Drug Administration (FDA) is responsible for regulating software applications that deal with medical care. The FDA requires that companies seek their clearance when an app behaves as a medical device and can potentially increase patient risk if the app does not work properly. Examples of apps that have sought and received FDA clearance include Diabetes Logbook by mySugr GmbH, AliveECG from AliveCor, and Propeller Health (for COPD and asthma management). In these cases, an app links to the medical device, such as a glucometer for measuring blood glucose or an inhaler for respiratory disease management.

Use of mobile health apps can support patient discussions with physicians and encourage shared decision-making: four in ten people who used health apps also discussed or shared mobile app data with their doctor. The most common mHealth apps "prescribed" or recommended by physicians to patients in 2015 were MyFitnessPal's Calorie Counter, Lose It!, QuitSTART (for smoking cessation), Map My Fitness workout trainer, and Every Body Walk!, developed by Kaiser Permanente.[275]

While wearable tech for health and wellness started with digital pedometers activated with accelerometer sensors, newer devices are fitted with several sensors to multi-task tracking of more than one function. The 2019 CES featured devices that went well beyond steps and activity to include tracking of heart function, stress levels, air quality and calories in food.[276]

Smartwatches are becoming a new-and-improved breed of watch just as smartphones have largely replaced texting phones. By 2021, more than one-third of watches sold will be smartwatches, capable of enabling mobile payments, notifications, voice functions, and health and wellness apps.[277]

Tracking and wearable technologies are going well beyond the wrist, which, since the advent of the Fitbit in 2007, has been the most popular body site for consumer wearable tech. Devices on the market can be worn, literally, from head to toe.

The growing evidence on connecting for health

Improving patient outcomes and better managed healthcare costs are proof of the growing value of using digital health tools.[278] If digital health apps were broadly used with just five conditions and/or programs– diabetes prevention, diabetes care, asthma, cardiac rehabilitation, and pulmonary rehabilitation – the U.S. healthcare system could save as much as $7 billion a year.

IQVIA, a clinical research and analytics company, reviewed hundreds of studies focusing on Type 2 diabetes, depression and anxiety. At least 860 clinical trials using digital health tools were in process in 2017, employing text messaging and home-based remote monitoring. Based on the research, design and "stickiness" (sustained use) of digital health tools were improving.

Barriers remain when it comes to consumers' digital health adoption. How are patients to choose from among the thousands of choices available in app stores? Could app "formularies" help, which would be curated by physicians who have prescribed and tracked patient use of various digital health tools? Who pays for the digital health tools? How can patient privacy be ensured as data flows from consumer health devices which may not be covered by HIPAA regulations, to the patient's electronic health record and to potentially other third party databases that may fall outside of HIPAA provisions? (See the next chapter for a deeper discussion on health data privacy.)

Wearing, tracking health

CES 2019 featured wearable tech for health and medical care on a continuum from tracking activity and sleep using a fashionable, customizable Move watch from Withings priced at $69 (and made in America), to gauging blood pressure at the wrist through the FDA-cleared Omron HeartGuide watch initially marketed at $499.

Most Americans track some aspect of their health, commonly monitoring their weight, blood pressure, food intake (calories, nutrition), steps, and exercise. In 2017, tracking health and fitness ranked highest among all reasons to buy wearable devices. Consumers using wearable tech are also tracking other people (for example, aging parents living at home, or children's activity), and even their pets' wellness.

For tracking health, wearable tech is a growing category including health and fitness bands, smartwatches, AR/VR headsets, smart clothing, and biometric sensors. In 2016, just one in four people used wearable devices to track health. Wearable tech adoption is expected to reach critical mass by 2021, according to Forrester Research.[279] With over 7 percent growth rate in the third quarter of 2017, Fitbit, Xiaomi, and Apple were the top suppliers for wearable tech at that time.[280]

With health and fitness ranking high on consumer's shopping lists,[281] it is not surprising that retailers like Walmart and Best Buy along with retail pharmacies are trusted channels for wearable health products.[282] Walgreens has grown its loyalty program, Balance Rewards, by enabling consumers' to earn points by using their trackers; those points can then be spent in the retailer's stores and online portal. Beyond shopping discounts, this kind of program has the potential to enhance a patient's continuity of care by sharing real-time data to improve health. It also encourages consumers to keep using the tracking devices since they are so closely linked to short term rewards.

Wearing your digital health on your sleeve

Sonny Vu, founder of Misfit Wearables (acquired by the Fossil Group in 2015, and then by Google in early 2019), believes that activity tracking shouldn't need a dedicated device to do the work: he sees a future where sensors will be built into your favorite t-shirt, a cap, a belt, or in shoes.[283] His company's device The Shine launched in 2012 and was designed as a stainless steel disc that could be worn anywhere: on the wrist, around the neck encased in a pendant, or carried in a pocket.

Wearables for health are evolving to include clothing embedded with sensors incorporated into fabrics, referred to as smart textiles or e-textiles. Vu's future vision of smart clothing has been available for the athletic and sports markets, in shirts (e.g., Zephyr) and shoes (e.g., Nike+ Lebron X) regularly used by athletes. Smart textiles are being further developed for medical uses, such as monitoring patients recovering from surgery where sensors measure vital signs such as blood pressure, heart rate, muscle exertion, and skin conductivity.

The iconic Levi's denim jacket was first sold in 1967. Known as the Type III Commuter Trucker jacket, a new model was launched to celebrate its 50th birthday in 2017.[284] Levi's collaborated with Project Jacquard from Google's Advanced Technology and Projects (ATAP) division. Project Jacquard's tagline is, "with a literal brush of your cuff, you can navigate your life while living it." The jacket was woven with a conductive threat that enabled communication with a hardware platform allowing the wearer to communicate via calls and texts without touching a phone; navigate, get the time, and estimated time of arrival; and, listen to music.

Nanowear, which develops medical-grade smart textiles, received FDA clearance in 2016 for its SimplECG garment: the fabric is embedded with sensors and couple with an app that captures continuous multi-channel ECG, heart rate, and respiratory rate data communicating to a portal for review by a physician or health coach.[285] The company's vision is to be part of a connected health system that ensures continuity of care, especially for patients managing chronic conditions such as heart disease, which can benefit from continuous monitoring.

Digital therapeutics – software as medicine

Digital therapeutics complement traditional treatments like medications (which McKinsey calls "digital companions") or as digital tools to substitute for prescription drugs.[286]

In 2010, the WellDoc BlueStar device was cleared by the FDA as the first prescription medical technology to help consumers manage type 2 diabetes. BlueStar was the first instance of an FDA-cleared digital health tool designed for doctors to prescribe to consumers for use at home. The technology can be prescribed by healthcare providers with the goal of patients' better managing their care at home, outside of the doctor's office, based on real-time transmission of blood glucose data. The data is transmitted to WellDoc's analytics system, which analyzes the data and coaches the patient with education and medication management advice. In January 2017, WellDoc received another clearance for a consumer-grade BlueStar digital therapeutic to be sold over-the-counter, with no prescription necessary.

WellDoc's pioneering work led the way for digital therapeutics, which deliver medicine in the form of software. Prescription digital therapeutics (PDTs) are clinically-proven, FDA-cleared software applications that are shown to be safe and effective in clinical trials to improve patient outcomes. They are meant to enhance clinical outcomes in combination with current treatments provided through drug and medical devices. PDTs can take the form of patient-facing applications, outcomes tracking, clinician monitoring tools, and HIPAA-compliant data storage.

In September 2017, the FDA cleared a prescription digital therapeutic (PDT) to treat substance use disorders related to abuse of alcohol, illicit and prescription drugs. Pear Therapeutics' product, reSET, is a 12-week cognitive behavioral therapy program used in conjunction with standard outpatient treatment for substance use disorder to treat misuse of alcohol, cannabis, cocaine, and stimulants. Clinical trial data for this PDT showed that one-half of patients who used the app abstained from using substances for three months versus 17.6 percent of patients who used standard therapy alone.

The Digital Therapeutics Alliance, a group of industry stakeholders, came together in late 2017 to promote the adoption and use of the innovations in mainstream healthcare. The Alliance's initial members included Alili Interactive, Omada Health, Pear Therapeutics, Propeller Health, Voluntis, and WellDoc. It is important to note that not all digital therapeutics undergo FDA regulatory scrutiny, and thus aren't referred to formally as "prescriptions."

Telehealth and virtual care

In 1962, "Uniblab" was episode ten in the cartoon series *The Jetsons*, in which Jane and George Jetson's son Elroy was unwell.

To tend to her son's care, Jane called up the doctor on the family's videophone screen.[287]

Nearly six decades later, telehealth, the use of electronic and telecommunications technologies to deliver clinical health services,[288] fulfills our consumer demand to access health care services right here, right now. "Here" can be home, at work on our smartphones, or in a virtual health kiosk at the grocery store or retail pharmacy. As long as there is a broadband connection between the patient and provider, telehealth technology can deliver care at anytime, anywhere.

Telehealth is a broad umbrella of applications that can deliver health services virtually: via live (real-time), two-way interaction between a person and provider; non-real time (referred to as "asynchronous"), secure e-mail, allowing the provider to review a patient's information, consider it, and provide feedback (say, a diagnosis or prescription); remote patient monitoring (RPM), where a person collects data generated by wearable technology (e.g., a wristband), a biometric device (such as a digital glucometer to measure blood glucose for diabetes tracking), or other clinical sensors (say, a digital blood pressure cuff), which collect and communicate data to a provider who can track patients' conditions and provide feedback for ongoing care; and, mobile technology, enabling text messaging with medication reminders and healthy behavior nudges.

The more people have been exposed to telehealth, the more likely consumers will expect it to be bundled into routine care delivery. Most consumers are interested in seeing their primary care doctor over video; parents with younger children under 18 would be especially keen to have their doctors (namely, pediatricians) offer telehealth. One in five people would switch from their current primary care doctor to one that offers telehealth visits, an American Well survey found.[289]

In addition to convenience, a telehealth visit can be significantly less expensive than a traditional doctor's visit. In one study comparing costs in 2016, an ER visit averaged $1,572; an urgent care visit, $163; a visit to a primary care provider, $142; a retail clinic visit, $88. In contrast, American Well offered a virtual visit for $49 that year direct-to-consumer.

These large cost differences have also motivated employers to offer telehealth as an employee benefit as part of health insurance programs. In 2018, two-thirds of U.S. companies offered a telemedicine benefit as part of their health plan.[290] Health insurance companies have also begun to reimburse telehealth services, and Medicare is now covering virtual healthcare for specific uses. Coverage of telehealth has become a go-to tactic for managing ever-increasing workplace health insurance costs, nudging workers to lower-cost settings like telehealth for both medical and mental health care.[291]

With the goal of keeping patients affiliated with their health systems and driving efficiencies to lower costs, other health care providers are adopting telehealth with the aim of extending the hospital walls into peoples' communities. The Mercy Virtual Care Center in Missouri was built as a hospital without beds: everything that happens in the Center is virtual. Consumers who want to access Mercy Virtual's services use a personal digital health device at home (such as a Wi-Fi enabled blood pressure monitor or weight scale) and stream the vital sign data to the Mercy Virtual "command center." Clinicians observe the patient data over time and can intervene when they perceive a change in a person's health status. By 2017, Mercy Virtual was serving over 600,000 patients living in eight states.[292]

Kaiser Permanente conducts over one-half of patient visits virtually through video visits, telephone, and secure messaging (HIPAA-compliant e-mail). Sixty percent of visits to KP.org are done from a mobile device.[293]

Kaiser has proven that telehealth and virtual visits can work well among a diverse group of patients, from younger to older, and across a broad variety ethnically and culturally varied people that the health system serves. That's on the "supply," or provider, side of telehealth.

On the demand side, nearly all patients believe they are personally in charge of their own health and care.[294] Combine that mass market sense of self-health empowerment with the ethos of "I want what I want when I want it" (the Amazon Prime effect), and you get a sense of peoples' pent-up demand for virtual health services.

In this emerging era of telehealth care, most consumers are interested in doing many health care tasks virtually, such as tracking health status (eg., blood glucose, blood pressure, pulse rate), having a follow-up appointment after seeing a doctor or other clinician, getting follow-up care at home after being discharged from hospital, getting reminders to do things to stay healthy, and getting daily support to manage an ongoing health issue.[295]

Telehealth at retail

Retail telehealth is offered direct-to-consumer through pharmacies and grocery stores, and through many employer benefit plans. CVS allies with several telehealth companies to channel virtual healthcare to consumers. Walgreens provides telehealth services

THE MAJORITY OF CONSUMERS ARE WILLING TO USE DIGITALLY ENABLED HEALTH CARE TECHNOLOGIES AT HOME

How likely are you to do the following?

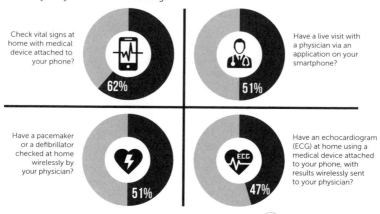

Check vital signs at home with medical device attached to your phone? **62%**

Have a live visit with a physician via an application on your smartphone? **51%**

Have a pacemaker or a defibrillator checked at home wirelessly by your physician? **51%**

Have an echocardiogram (ECG) at home using a medical device attached to your phone, with results wirelessly sent to your physician? **47%**

Source: Top health industry issues of 2019: The New Health Economy comes of age, PwC, Dec. 2018

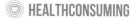

via their mobile app and website, and launched Walgreens Find Care in 2018 as a digital marketplace that connects Walgreens app users to doctors affiliated with both hospital systems throughout the U.S. as well as telehealth companies and Walgreens Healthcare Clinics, Hearing, and Optical professionals.[296]

Walmart piloted a walk-in telemedicine clinic in Houston in 2008. Ten years later, Walmart launched a program with telehealth provider Doctor on Demand and supplier Reckitt-Benckiser (RB), which markets the over-the-counter brands Airborne and Mucinex. With the purchase of an RB product, Walmart shoppers were offered a free telehealth visit with a board-certified physician from Doctor on Demand. "This initiative is a big first step in delivering on RB and Walmart's shared purpose of unlocking every American's right to healthier lives...Walmart shoppers are looking for new ways to take health matters into their own hands," Gregory Chabidon, CMO USA, RB Health Unit, said in the project's press release.[297] Walmart also launched a tele-mental health initiative with Beacon to provide accessible mental healthcare to veterans suffering from depression or PTSD.

BayCare Health System, a Tampa-Bay based hospital group, has partnered with 26 Publix pharmacies in their target market. BayCare-branded kiosks are in private rooms in the grocery stores, where shoppers-*cum*-patients can communicate with BayCare health providers about whatever health issues are on their mind.[298]

One of the most prevalent health kiosks enabling virtual visits is higi, with at least 11,000 devices located in over 50 grocery chains, Big Box stores, and pharmacies throughout the U.S. Three-quarters of the U.S. population lives within five miles of a higi retail location.[299] Using higi, consumers can conduct self-screening health tests for blood pressure, pulse, BMI, and weight. With their installed base of 52 million users, higi estimates the company performs about one million health screenings every week under HIPAA-compliant protocols. If consumers opt-in, higi also integrates data people generate through their activity trackers and mobile health apps, building out their health profile in the higi data ecosystem. To enable data integration between kiosks and hospitals' electronic health records, higi partners with Bridge Connector as data integrator.[300]

The growing role of Apple in health

Since apps launched in the Apple iTunes store in 2008, health has been a popular theme for consumer downloads. At the start, health apps focused on fitness and lifestyle, with food tracking, exercise and weight management among the most downloaded mobile tools. Bolstering its consumer brand equity, Apple aligned with some of the most popular health and wellness brands at the time, such as Nike, Mayo Clinic, and WebMD.

Apple enjoys consumer brand-love for its phones and computers, and is globally admired for strong brand equity.[301] At Apple's shareholder meeting held in February 2018, CEO Tim Cook told investors he was looking to build brand-love for consumer health, as well, stating, "We're in this really great position that we can do what we've always done, which is look at it as the user looks at it... We can ask ourselves, how can we improve the health of the user, not worrying about if we can convince the federal government to give us a reimbursement or not. This is an area Apple can make serious contributions over time."[302]

In early 2018, Apple's health website landing page asserted that, "The future of healthcare is in your hands."[303] After months in stealth mode, Apple publicly announced they were working with a dozen major healthcare providers on deploying electronic health records to the iPhone Health app. Based on the list of providers, it was clear that Apple was making a major commitment to break into the EHR space, long dominated by "big iron" players like Cerner, Epic, and Allscripts. That initial list included some of the most wired health IT users, among them Johns Hopkins Medicine, Cedars-Sinai, Penn Medicine, Geisinger Health System, Rush University Medical Center, and the Ochsner Health System.[304]

Central to Apple's healthcare strategy is its emerging role in patient/person-centered electronic health records. In 2016, Apple acquired Gliimpse, a platform for consumers allowing them to aggregate and share their personal health data.[305]

By April 2018, Apple was collaborating with at least 40 health systems on deploying patients' health records to their phones.[306]

Apple's large installed consumer base could be key to the

company's ability to scale healthcare. Apple's base of iPhone users in the U.S. topped 86 million in 2018; Anthem, the health plan, had 40 million members, and UnitedHealthcare, 50 million enrollees.

One of the first studies that ResearchKit supported focused on heart disease with researchers at Stanford University School of Medicine.[307] Within 24 hours of Stanford launching the MyHeart Counts app for the study, to study heart health, 11,000 people had signed up to participate. "To get 10,000 people enrolled in a medical study normally, it would take a year and 50 medical centers around the country," Dr. Alan Yeung, medical director of Stanford Cardiovascular Health, told Bloomberg. "That's the power of the phone."[308]

Not just any phone: Dr. Yeung was referring to the iPhone that served as all the patients' research platform for participating in the study.

We can expect the iPhone and Apple Watch to be growing platforms for both consumer health and medical care. Consumers can access clinical lab tests results from LabCorp and Quest, as well as conduct an EKG test using Apple products for which developers have innovated applications for ophthalmology, diabetes, orthopedics, audiology, and cardiology.[309] The company's growing list of medical patents and hiring of professionals from every aspect of the healthcare ecosystem suggest that "saying Aaaaaaaple" may be the next incarnation of saying "ahhhh."[310]

Welcome to the Internet of Things for health at home

"By 2020, everything we build at Samsung will be connected to the Internet," forecasted B.K. Yoon, CEO of Samsung, in a keynote speech at the 2015 CES.[311]

Imagine a world where your home nurtures your health and wellness. If you develop a chronic illness, where you live will be your care-giving hub. Home appliances and your bathroom and bed will know you, and your kitchen will anticipate your preferences and feed your health based on your medical needs and taste profile.

That world is fast-evolving. Increasingly, these "things" will be used by patients, consumers and caregivers for health and medical care at home, away from the bricks-and-mortar of hospitals, physician offices, and outpatient clinics.

Within a few weeks in early 2015, three meetings convened that hinted the start of the Internet of Things for health: the CES, focusing on consumer tech; HIMSS, the annual mega-meeting of healthcare providers and technology geeks who design, buy, implement, and use healthcare information technology in hospitals and doctors' offices; and, South-by-Southwest (SXSW), the interactive conference in Austin that also features music movies, technology.

One vendor showed at all three conferences: Philips. At the time, the company had doubled-down on digital health and divested the company of assets that didn't touch health or healthcare, like hospital-based MRI and CT scanners and inpatient monitors, or maternal and fetal monitors for pregnant women. For decades, Philips had been a major supplier of digital health technologies in medical care; increasingly, the company was expanding its product portfolio for peoples' health at home, from the baby's nursery to the kitchen and safe aging-in-place. At CES 2015, the company made a big splash about health-at-home; at HIMSS, consolidating the company's position in digital imaging and population health; and, at SXSW, handing out healthy smoothies made by Philips blenders in food trucks adjacent to the Austin Convention Center.

That's when the green shoots of the Internet of Things for health at home emerged for mainstream consumers.

Philips' vision of the smart nursery was an early entrant to the Internet of Things (IoT) for a healthy home: think, "The Internet of Baby." By 2017, most parents said they would buy into the IoT, whether a smart TV or a baby health tracking device. A BabyCenter survey of parents with children found that IoT devices – such as connected cars, health and fitness tracking devices, smart baby and children's toys, and smart kitchen appliances – helped parents make lives easier and made them feel like better parents.[312] The most popular connected devices owned by these parents included smart TVs, streaming TV devices (like Apple TV or Roku), health and fitness tracking devices (such as Fitbit), and smart baby and children's toys. The top motivation of parents for acquiring IoT devices were to make life easier, save time, have more control, have the newest technology, and for safety and security.

The Internet of Healthy Things, as Dr. Joseph Kvedar of the Center for Connected Health has coined the phenomenon, covers connected devices to help people manage health and wellness as well as disease and illness in the home.[313]

The most common health metric that people track is weight.[314] Ponder the role of a connected weight scale in the landscape of the Internet of Medical Things. A scale is useful, first, for overall wellness, to track weight. If the device has advanced features, it might detect fat pounds versus overall weight and calculate a body mass index (BMI), and heart function. Over time, knowing these numbers can play a helpful role in helping people achieve and subsequently manage a weight goal. (Consider that 70 percent of people in the U.S. were overweight or obese in 2015).[315]

Now think about the value that a connected scale can play to help a patient dealing with congestive heart failure (CHF). One of the most important metrics a CHF patient must track is weight, to watch for water retention; if a patient's weight increases by just a few pounds over a few days, the rise can mean greater risk for hospitalization, perhaps preceded by a fall at home.

If a medical practice connects with the weight data generated by the scale, with the opting-in permission of the patient, a nurse or health coach can intervene with the patient before a fall or emergency room admission. The clinician can recommend increasing a dose of a diuretic or other medication; initiate a virtual visit over a smartphone, tablet, or PC; or, ask the patient to come directly to the office for a face-to-face visit.

The connected bathroom for health and wellness

As weight scales sold to consumers at retail are increasingly connected devices, so, too, will be other items used in our bathrooms, which are important hubs of health and wellness. CareOS, an operating system of standards for the connected bathroom, exhibited at CES 2018. Their booth was crowded by media and health industry stakeholders who were curious to learn about a smart mirror platform for a connected bathroom. "CareOS takes care of you" was the project's tag-line, which envisions augmented reality and artificial intelligence connecting devices for the smart bathroom.

At CES 2018, that prototype bathroom was a softly lit, spa-green environment placed in the midst of the hard-tech context of CES. CareOS is fostering the standards for the connected bathroom, partnering with organizations in the health and beauty ecosystem: at CES, they announced partnerships with Hydrao, with an eco-friendship shower; iHealth, with health monitoring tools including a digital scale and diabetes apps; Kaertech, which develops connected objects; Kolibree, maker of a connected toothbrush; PlumeLabs, with a focus on air quality; Radioline, a digital radio service; Romy Paris, a skin care company; Skinjay, a bathroom supplier; Snips, a voice assistant developer; Tefal, whose personal care division is working with CareOS; Terraillon's personal wellbeing group; and, Tucky, featuring connected baby products.

At the group's launch at CES 2018, CareOS met with interested retailers, hotel chains, long-term care companies, health insurance plans, hair salon groups and big beauty players. While a new concept to these organizations, the connected bathroom represents a potentially impactful health hub for digitized personal care.

Skin cancer is the most common form of cancer in the United States.[316] Over five million cases of non-melanoma skin cancer were treated in over 3 million people in the U.S. in 2012.[317] One in five Americans will develop skin cancer by the age of 70.[318]

Imagine that you had a smart mirror in your bathroom which could take 4D visualizations, resulting in pictures of you on all sides of your body, including your back. If you found a spot, you could track it over time and, if the image visibly changed, then share it with your doctor. In so doing, this application enables a channel for tele-dermatology between patient and doctor.

Beyond the utility of a connected bathroom, from managing weight to spotting a suspicious mole, the issue of privacy is paramount — particularly in this most private space in one's home. "We have to be able to lock CareOS," Chloe Szulzinger, Director of Communications for the project, told me. "It's a closed secure network in the same way that in the bathroom, you can lock the door," she explained.

CareOS was developed along Privacy by Design (PbD) principles, a framework that proactively embeds privacy into the design and operation of IT systems, networks, and business practices.[319] At its core, PbD supports the view that privacy assurance must become an organization's default mode of operation, applied with "special vigor to sensitive data such as medical information," Ann Cavoukian wrote in the 7 Foundational Principles of PbD.

Based on the CareOS's commitment to PbD, the OS works with the WiFi in a home, using two chips to protect personal data. "Nothing can go directly from CareOS to Instagram," Szulzinger explained.

In the connected bathroom, as Amazon's Alexa calls up, say, your Kohler Verdura smart mirror, you could also start your car via Alexa while finishing up your tooth-brushing or weigh-in.

Your car – a "third space" for health

The IoT for health, enabled through Alexa and other voice-assistants, will extend beyond the phone and household appliances, bathrooms and bedrooms. Your car will be a third space for health, after home (the first space) and work (the second space).

In 2016, Nissan sponsored a research study into the future car industry in Europe, titled "Freeing the Road: Shaping the Future for Autonomous Vehicles." Beyond many economic benefits cited in favor of autonomous cars, health benefits could include a reduction of driver stress and car accidents that lead to trauma and, at worst, mortality.[320] Mobile health (mHealth) has been long defined as care delivered via mobile communications platforms, such as smartphones and tablets. Think of the car as the third space for health, literally enabling mobile health.

Hyundai presented a prototype mobile health scenario at CES 2017 as the Health + Mobility Cockpit. The concept car was embedded with sensors, designed to read the driver's levels of stress and alertness. Lighting, scents (à la aromatherapy), and other tailored "mood bursts" would be deployed based on the sensors' readings: for example, if a driver wasn't perceived to be alert, a peppermint scent might be released in the car as an energy-boost. A stressed driver might inhale eucalyptus or lavender.

We can expect health and wellness to be delivered in our autos as an extension of home health: Fiat Chrysler's Portal envisioned a seamless connection between our homes and workplaces.[321]

Marry the Internet of Healthy Things at home to a car and you might envision a self-driving auto that makes house calls.[322] A concept called Aim, developed by design firm Artefact, brought together connected home elements for health, like the smart bathroom and connected kitchen with wearable technology to bolster the continuum of healthcare embodied in a self-driving clinic. The vision is that all of these devices collect data about us that, together, could reveal an underlying health condition or acute event, like a predicted high-risk for falling or dramatically elevated blood sugar, based on AI. When that data point is revealed, a self-driving car would be dispatched home to check in with you.

The emergence and importance of electronic health records

Consumers expect the health care system – doctors, hospitals, pharmacies, and other providers – to use computers the way other industries they deal with in daily life do, like banks and grocery stores. The use of electronic health records by health care providers has grown with the financial nudging (incentive payments) from American taxpayers embodied in the Health Information Technology for Economic and Clinical Health Act (HITECH). HITECH was part of the economic stimulus bill, the American Recovery and Reinvestment Act of 2009 (ARRA), which preceded and laid the groundwork for enactment of the Affordable Care Act the following year.

As part of the stimulus bill, HITECH was effectively a stimulus for the adoption and effective use of electronic records by doctors and hospitals in the U.S. The Act allocated $35 billion to encourage adoption of EHRs by healthcare providers in the U.S. by 2014. Before HITECH, only 42 percent of physicians had an EHR in their office, with most doctors keeping patients' medical records in paper files and cabinets.[323] In 2016, over 90 percent of both U.S. hospitals and doctors had installed an EHR.[324,325]

Doctors' and hospitals' use of EHRs have many benefits for patients, improving coordination of care and health outcomes. The lag of health information technology use in the U.S. compromised safety, efficiency and effectiveness of health care for every health citizen in the country. *Paper Kills* was the title of a book with a forward by Newt Gingrich published in 2007, highlighting how personal health information stored in paper-based folders and file cabinets could lead to medical errors, inefficiency and privacy breaches.[326]

In 2005, Hurricane Katrina was a wake-up call for the healthcare industry when it came to digitizing patient records.[327] The storm virtually erased the paper medical records of thousands of Gulf Coast residents. "We don't want people to be saved, taken to a shelter and then face the risk of death because doctors don't know what's going on with them," Dr. David Brailer, then national coordinator for health information technology at the Department of Health and Human Services, said. Newt Gingrich's observation following Katrina was that, "Paper records are an utterly irrational national security risk."

Beyond this catastrophic risk, EHRs potentially enable people to access personal health information (PHI) on a 24×7 basis; avoid duplicate tests; enhance patient safety and improve medication management to avoid adverse events (e.g., overdosing, hazardous mixing of medications, drug-drug interactions); enable secure communication of patient data between health providers (say, a primary care doctor to a specialist) to better coordinate care; and, avoid ineligible handwriting when the doctor writes a prescription or follow-up instructions.

Many of these benefits were identified in an important report published in 2001, *Crossing the Quality Chasm*, published by the Institute of Medicine.[328] This report called out the faults in the U.S. health system that were risks for patient safety, equity and efficiency – all of which were addressed in some way in the Affordable Care Act and the HITECH Act.

Ironically and significantly, EHRs themselves can present risks when they are poorly designed and implemented. Fortune magazine and Kaiser Health News published "Death by a Thousand Clicks," an investigative report documenting many cases where digital health records had contributed to a patient's death or disability.[329] The authors uncovered many risks attributable to EHRs. One week before the story was printed, ECRI Institute curated their top ten patient safety concerns of 2019; number one was, "diagnostic stewardship and test result management using EHRs."[330]

The Fortune/Kaiser team reported, "patient deaths, serious injuries, and near misses...tied to software glitches, user errors, or other flaws" in both public and private-sector systems. The errors were documented in the largest EHRs used by academic medical centers as well as smaller systems that have been adopted in community hospitals. While the authors pointed out that medical errors were rife in paper-based medical files, the mistakes emerging from the digitization of medical records embodied unintended consequences of moving medical records out of the filing cabinet and into digital formats. The growing epidemic of physician burnout has also led to some doctors blaming EHRs, as doctors have been forced to devote several hours a day just to deal with poorly designed digital health records.

The "e" in "EHR" can mean "empowered"

When well-conceived, co-designed with health care providers and users, and effectively implemented, data accessed from EHRs can give people a sense of control over their health. Viewing digital health records empowered patients and their caregivers in a study of people using MyHealtheVet, the EHR system of the Veterans Administration Health System. Patients felt seeing their records enhanced communication with health providers and peoples' ability to self-care at home, along with participating in shared medical decision making with their doctors.[331]

People who gain access to their EHR online can become inspired to ask their doctors more questions and share in decision-making. A study sponsored by California Healthcare Foundation found that when patients with lower-incomes, multiple chronic conditions, and/or advanced age were given access to their EHRs, the patients became more engaged with their personal health information and asked physicians more questions about their health conditions and treatment options.[332]

Most patients who have accessed their EHRs said computer use in the exam room improved their quality of care, and felt their clinician was more aware of their medical history. Furthermore, most patients whose doctors used an EHRs rated the quality of their care excellent compared with patients whose doctors did not use an EHR.[333]

Another study found patients whose doctors used EHRs were less likely to sue them for malpractice. Major risk factors for malpractice claims include poor communication between doctors and patients, difficulty in accessing patient information in a timely manner, unsafe prescribing practices, and lower adherence to clinical guidelines – all of which can be addressed through EHRs and computer-based medical records.[334]

OpenNotes and OurNotes

Despite the advent of EHRs, there's a component in a person's health record that's traditionally been a no-patient's-land: the physician's notes, which have traditionally been off-limits to patients' eyes.

Transparency in health care can bring greater empowerment and enable more rational decision making for health consumers. There's evidence that patients will embrace transparency in the form of accessing their physicians' notes about them, based on the OpenNotes project.[335]

The original OpenNotes study measured the impact on doctors and patients of extending patients access to view their doctors' notes over a secure Internet portal. The trial was done at three medical centers: Beth Israel Deaconess Medical Center in Massachusetts, Geisinger Health System in Pennsylvania, and Harborview Medical Center in Washington state, where thousands of patients and over 100 physicians were involved in the study.

Virtually all patients involved wanted to continue to have access to doctor's notes, a significant finding. However, even more powerful was that most patients wanted to be able to add comments to doctors' notes, which one-third of doctors said would also be useful.

A majority of patients agreed that OpenNotes could have many benefits for them, including taking better care of themselves, better understanding health conditions, remembering care plans, more effectively preparing for visits, and feeling more in control of their care.

Most physicians agreed that nothing was difficult about the OpenNotes program and they experienced no changes in their practice (such as workflow interruptions and productivity loss).

For those patients who want to engage with their health more actively, the OpenNotes project gives credence to the fact that patients *can* handle the truth. Reading one's physician notes is a fundamental step in a patient's transformational journey toward empowerment. The OpenNotes researchers pointed to a quote from a patient focus group: "Having it written down, it's almost like there's another person telling you to take your meds."

By 2018, about 21 million people had access to their doctor's notes through online portals. With that level of patient traction, OpenNotes is evolving into the OurNotes project, an effort that will allow patients to add comments about their healthcare concerns and observations that might otherwise not be articulated in the exam room in real-time.[336] "This is an invitation to get the patient to contribute more and set the agenda for talking to their doctor," Dr. John Mafi at the David Geffen School of Medicine at UCLA believes.[337]

As patients share their health experiences with doctors, people are increasingly sharing their data with researchers and other patients, as well.

Sharing data and data altruism

Generating data isn't enough. It also needs to be shared to make it valuable. As Stanford's Apple ResearchKit study found, people are willing to share their personal health data...on their own terms. Consumers have decidedly different opinions on who to trust for sharing their health data. Most consumers are open to sharing data with doctors, insurance companies, and pharmacies; only a minority of people would share with pharmaceutical companies, government agencies, or tech companies.[338]

A *Consumer Reports* survey concurred with this research, with 9 in 10 people agreeing that their health data should be used to help improve the care of future patients who might have the same or similar condition.[339]

PatientsLikeMe launched their Data for Good campaign in 2014, marking a decade as one of the first online patient social networks. The site was founded by the Heywood brothers who built an online platform to help a third brother deal with ALS. Promoting the Data for Good project in a YouTube video, Jamie Heywood explained, "The one person, you, who is living with the thing that has changed your life, you're not really part of the process. Medicine doesn't understand illness. It doesn't understand how treatments are used in the real world. What it's like to walk a mile in a patient's shoes. The dream that we are working on is to take your experience and turn it into something that gives you a real voice to make the system about you the patient." PatientsLikeMe brings together people dealing with dozens of conditions, all contributing their data in the community. These data are then shared with researchers at institutions and companies to better inform discoveries.

As Ed, a PatientsLikeMe member managing Parkinson's Disease, attested on the video, "We can do much better fighting the disease

CONSUMERS WITH A CHRONIC CONDITION ARE MORE WILLING TO SHARE THEIR TRACKED DATA

Survey question: How willing would you be to share the information tracked in your apps or devices for the following reasons?*

	CHRONIC DESEASE	NO CHRONIC DESEASE	TOTAL
Blinded/anonymous contribution to an organization that does health care research	43%	34%	39%
Blinded/anonymous contribution to a device developer to improve device/program	44%	34%	40%
Share with emergency services if experiencing a sudden emergency situation	58%	46%	53%
Alert myself and share with family if in danger due to a fall or other health emergency situation	57%	48%	53%
Share with my doctors to help them provide better care to me	66%	52%	60%

*Chart shows the percentage of respondents who answered 4 or 5 on a 5-point scale, where 1 is "not at all willing" and 5 is "extremely willing."

Note: For the purposes of this research, a "chronic condition" is defined as any disease or health problem that has lasted for three or more months. Examples include arthritis, diabetes, cancer, heart disease, high blood pressure, high cholesterol, asthma, allergies, back pain, depression, alcohol or drug dependence, and others. Source: Deloitte 2018 Survey of US Health Care Consumers.

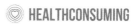 **HEALTHCONSUMING**

as a group than we can as individuals."[340] This demonstrates the concept of data altruism—the idea of paying it forward for other patients and families by sharing one's own data.

When people are sick or dealing with a chronic health condition, they are more willing to share the data tracked in their devices and apps.[341] Most people with chronic disease say they would share their health data with doctors to help them provide better care, and a plurality of patients would also share data with a device developer; a plurality of patients would also share data with a device developer to improve that tracking tool.

Consumers also willingly share data with loyalty programs, such as Walgreens Balance Rewards. The program enables Walgreens shoppers who opt-in to link their fitness and medical tracking devices to the app, earning points that can be used as dollars for shopping in the store. By 2018, Balance Rewards linked to 38 devices and 24 health apps, including the Apple Watch as well as Walgreens' own branded activity tracker, Striiv.[342]

Peer-to-peer healthcare

For health, "your community is your superpower," as Susannah Fox, a noted data sharing advocate and former U.S. Health and Human Services Chief Technology Officer has asserted.[343]

Fox has been gathering evidence on patients touching base with other patients online since she began to track the use of the Internet in healthcare for the Pew Research Group in the 2000s. Since then, the phenomenon of peer-to-peer (P2P) health support has grown.

While most health consumers use the internet to seek health information, there is a growing cadre of people who go online to find people with the same conditions they have, or to touch base with other caregivers experiencing similar situations. Social media enables people to be better health consumers by giving them peers' views on medical conditions, health products and health services in and outside of their physical and geographic communities.

"The Internet gives patients and caregivers access not only to information, but also to each other," observed Fox.

"The biggest motivator for health change is relationships," Margie Morris, a senior research scientist with Intel, learned through her research into people and their health behaviors.[344] Her ethnographic studies have found people to be highly motivated by the potential loss of social capital. In recognition of this, the Facebook-based app "A Little Health From My Friends" helps people stick with their health 'contracts' – agreements they make with others in their social network.

Using social networks for health is no longer a pioneering activity for bleeding-edge patient activists: Facebook has gone mainstream among patients and medical companies alike. A story in the July 2012 issue of *Good Housekeeping* magazine titled "Miracle on Facebook" shared the story of a family seeking a kidney for organ transplant for their 23-year old son, Ryan. Given a waiting list prospect of 3 years, Ryan's family took to the Internet and posted a video on Facebook about the need for a kidney donation. Ryan's mom had 200 Facebook friends who virally distributed the video through their networks. Within a few days, 10 people had stepped up to volunteer their organs to Ryan. Eventually, a relative of Ryan's mom, who had seen the video, donated her kidney and Ryan has recovered.

Tom Ferguson and Dan Hoch confirmed the power of P2P healthcare back in 2005 when they wrote,[345]

"Many patients are now ready, willing, and able to take a more active role in their own care, and the care of others with related diseases. By encouraging patients to do more for themselves and for each other, clinicians can help mitigate many of the negative effects of contemporary time-pressured medical practice. Thus, even though there may now be less time for the counseling, storytelling, support, information sharing, and empowerment-based training that was once a routine part of the typical office visit, we can now help our patients obtain such services by referring them to online patient networks."

To engage patients in more people-powered medical research, the Affordable Care Act (ACA), created the Patient Centered Outcomes Research Institute (PCORI). PCORI was founded on the concept that patients have values, preferences, opinions and concerns that are not always considered in traditional protocols for medical research. PCORI has funded research comparing treatments and health services that incorporates patients' and families' input. In 2015, the Institute had a $1.2 bn portfolio covering 468 projects in 41 states, studying mental/behavioral health, cancer, cardiovascular health, rare diseases, nutritional and metabolic disorders, among other conditions.[346] The FDA has also recognized the importance of patient-centered research and real-world evidence, encouraging and requiring that companies seeking their approval for products incorporate patient-reported outcomes into clinical trials.

The most ambitious patient-powered research program might be All of Us, launched by the U.S. National Institutes of Health. All of Us was designed to be the largest longitudinal research project with a goal of signing up at least one million U.S. participants to share data and prevent disease based on peoples' unique environment, genetics, and lifestyle.

Learning from Fred Holliday

Fred Holliday was diagnosed with metastatic kidney cancer on March 27, 2009. He was hospitalized several times. In April 2009, his wife, Regina asked one of the five hospitals in which Fred was a patient for a copy of his medical records so that she could learn the details of his condition, do research, and share in medical decision making.

The hospital's medical records department informed Regina that she could have a copy of Fred's records at a cost of 73 cents a page and a 21-day wait.

Fred died 82 days after he was diagnosed, on June 17, 2009.

When Regina ultimately got the copy of Fred's records, it was apparent that many mistakes were made and, while it's not clear that Fred's outcome would have changed, different decisions would likely have been made along the way. At that moment, Regina transformed into a patient advocate, evangelizing ever since about patient rights to data.

Americans' ability to access personal health information is a right under HIPAA, the Health Insurance Portability and Accountability Act. The acronym is often misunderstood: the "I" doesn't stand for "information" (it's for "insurance"), nor does the "P" represent "privacy" (that's for "portability").

Regina Holliday is not alone in her belief that people should be able to access their medical records. Most consumers believe they should have full access to their electronic health records, according to a 2016 Accenture survey.[347]

Peoples' ability to access personal health information can be a matter of life and death — and in between those two extremes on the continuum are quality of life, empowerment, and in the end, grace.

What if...Americans owned and controlled their medical and personal data, able to control, share and sell it based on personal opt-in and choice?

Chapter 6

PRIVACY AND HEALTH DATA IN-SECURITY

The growing problem of health data privacy and security

An employee of Med Center Health in Kentucky accessed 697,800 patient records, with details on diagnoses and procedure codes, health insurance information, Social Security numbers, and charges for medical services, resulting in the largest healthcare data breach in 2017.[348] The data thief intended to use the stolen health information for personal gain.

Nearly 4.4 million patient records were breached in the third quarter of 2018.[349] The number of breached records continued to climb quarter by quarter in 2018. One-half of these incidents were due to hacking, and one-fourth, by insider wrong-doing.

Nearly one-half of the ransomware incidents (aka cyber-extortion) that happened in 2017 occurred in healthcare.[350] The *per capita* cost of one breached medical record in America reached $408 in 2018, double the cost of a stolen record from banks.[351]

THE *PER CAPITA* COST OF DATA BREACH FOR HEALTH CARE IS FAR HIGHER THAN FOR OTHER INDUSTRIES

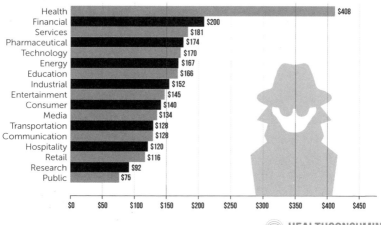

Source: The 2018 Cost of a Data Breach Study, Ponemon Institute and IBM Security, June 2018   ◎ HEALTHCONSUMING

The Office for Civil Rights as part of the federal Department of Health and Human Services (OCR) is responsible for the enforcement of the Health Insurance Portability and Accountability Act Privacy and Security Rules (HIPAA). While these rules have been enforceable since 2003, OCR has also been dealing with growing threats to Americans' personal health information among four types of bad actors:

- ◎ Nation-states, seeking economic, political, or military advantages
- ◎ Cyber-criminals, looking for financial gain
- ◎ Hacktivists, influencing political, social, and business change; and,
- ◎ Insiders, in search of personal advantage and monetary gain and/or professional revenge.[352]

While the external threats from hackers and cyber-criminals garner a lot of media coverage, insider threats are growing. Two-thirds of the threat actors in healthcare are internal.[353] An insider is anyone who has physical or remote access to personal health information via EHRs or other databases.

Healthcare is the only industry where employees are the predominant threat actors. Those threats can be malicious, with attackers seeking financial gain, which motivated two-thirds of the bad actors, or revenge.

The threat of external bad actors seeking to exploit personal health data is growing via ransomware and malware.[354] Eric Cowperthwaite, a security expert who led information security efforts at Providence Health & Services, was once warned about "nation state interest in health care." He believes that, "Health care, payers and providers both, are simply not prepared for the level of bad guy they are now facing."[355]

Medical records are very valuable relative to other breached consumer information. Personal health information has a longer "shelf-life" than other data (consider the longevity of a Social Security Number, for example). Furthermore, these breaches often don't get discovered for months. This makes stolen medical identities high-value for thieves to monetize.

Growing privacy awareness in America

Data privacy is now part of consumers' consciousness. Nine in 10 U.S. consumers believe it is important for companies to safeguard the privacy of their information.

In March 2017, former FBI Director James Comey asserted, "There is no such thing as absolute privacy in America."[356] Eighteen years before, in 1999, Scott McNealy, CEO of Sun Microsystems, presciently noted, "You have zero privacy anyway. Get over it."[357]

Americans are getting acclimatized to the growing risk-exposure of their personal data: one-half of U.S. adults don't trust the Federal government or social media sites to protect their data. [358]

Two-thirds of people in the U.S. were impacted by some sort of data theft, such as fraudulent charges on credit cards, notices that sensitive information (such as an account number) had been compromised, or an attempt by someone to take out credit in their name.

Personal information insecurity is now a fact of consumers' everyday life. One in two Americans feel their personal information is less secure now than it was five years ago.

The Equifax breach of 2017 profoundly changed Americans' views on data privacy. The incident impacted nearly 44 percent of the entire U.S. population. "This breach is a like a Category 5 hurricane in the cyberworld, affecting at least one-third of the U.S. population. The lasting impact from the breach will go on for years," forecasted Fleming Shi, a cybersecurity expert at Barracuda Networks.[359]

Most Americans don't believe their personal data is private and think companies should have to get permission before sharing or selling their online data, *Consumer Reports* learned in a survey conducted just months after President Donald Trump moved into the Oval Office.[360]

Consumers have grown less confident about both healthcare and data privacy, *Consumer Reports* found in their study on American sentiment conducted in the first half of 2017 – before the Equifax breach hit 143 million U.S. citizens. It's interesting to note that in the poll, CR assessed American perspectives covering both privacy *and* healthcare.

That study found that more Americans were growing pessimistic about their privacy rights and data protections based on the U.S. Congress's resolution changing (that is, weakening) FCC broadband privacy rules that required internet service providers to be required to get peoples' permission before selling or sharing consumers' data with other companies.

At the intersection of healthcare and privacy is the question of how much people value the security of their healthcare information (tied with what we say during our phone conversations). After one's Social Security Number, personal health information ranks second in a list of peoples' most sensitive data.[361]

The countervailing forces of trust and convenience

So who, then, do consumers trust with their personal data? For protecting data across-the-board, the number one trustworthy data steward among Americans is primary care doctors. At the bottom: governments, media and entertainment companies, and social media firms.[362]

But even as doctors are most-trusted to protect consumers' medical information, consumers remain concerned about the privacy of their electronic health records.[363]

"It depends" is the hedge-phrase that Americans use to characterize how people weigh their disclosure of personal information versus keeping private information private.

U.S. adults see a privacy trade-off, living in the convenience-context of the 21st century digital economy in exchange for some form of value. The "it depends" is a factor of what kind of data is getting collected, especially by third parties, how long the data are retained, for what use — *vis-à-vis* what a person is trading in return which could be a hard dollar value, convenience, knowledge, or support of some kind.

While one in four Americans say sharing health information is unacceptable under any conditions, another 20 percent say, "It depends."[364] Who remains is the one in two consumers who would be willing to share health information on a secure portal.

Overall, the "it depends" and privacy-absolutists are concerned about the following issues, which Pew gleaned through their survey:

- The initial bargain might be fine but the follow-up by companies that collect the data can be annoying and unwanted
- Scammers and hackers are a constant threat
- Location data seems especially precious in the age of the smartphone
- Profiling sometimes seems creepy (substitute "Big Brother" or "stalking" for "creepy").
- People are not happy when data are collected for one purpose but are used for other, often more invasive purposes.

The flip-side of these concerns are the potential benefits of personal data sharing, which include "free," a good price for, say, social media, email addresses, online storage, and other digital goodies; and, sharing can help "lubricate" commercial and social interactions.

Digital health tracking and the emergence of the digital phenotype

In 2017, the FDA cleared eighty-seven connected health devices that consumers could use continuous health monitoring. [365, 366] Diabetes, epilepsy, heart disease, dermatology, respiratory diseases, renal disease, neurological conditions, ophthalmology, and fertility were among the categories of devices cleared for patients' home use. This growing portfolio of medical devices can move care from provider settings to our homes.

With these advances come additional locations and occasions for clinical data to be created, outside of the hospital, clinic and doctor's office. These devices usually connect to a patient's smartphone through a Bluetooth and broadband connection and transmit data wirelessly to a medical record or other data destination.

When a patient using a remote health monitor transmits or stores that information with a HIPAA-covered entity – namely a hospital or physician – it becomes protected health information (PHI), subject to HIPAA Privacy and Security Rules. However, the data is not considered PHI when stored in the medical device itself.

In addition to people generating health data through wearable technology and remote health monitoring, people also leave "digital footprints" every day online.

I discussed this in a paper I wrote for the California Healthcare Foundation, *Here's Looking at You: How Personal Health Information Is Being Tracked and Used*. Consumer-created digital dust is being curated and collected, including peoples' Google health-related searches, participating in social networks, purchasing goods at retail (both online and in bricks-and-mortar stores), and passively communicating personal information like location via GPS sensors integrated into smartphones.[367]

"Our interactions with the digital world could actually unlock secrets of disease," Dr. Sachin Jain learned in work prior to taking his post as CEO of CareMore Health. CareMore embeds digital technology into its health system. The group has looked at Twitter to learn how tweets can show signs of sleep problems.[368]

Dr. Jain was referring to digital phenotyping, the concept that the data each individual generates on social media and digital devices can be combined and analyzed to provide insights into a patient. Dr. Jain collaborated with Dr. John Brownstein, Chief Innovation Office at Boston Children's Hospital, on a seminal article in *Nature Biotechnology* which explains the idea. Dr. Brownstein envisioned a growing role for this concept in individual and public health, explaining that, "Through social media, forums and online communities, wearable technologies and mobile devices, there is a growing body of health-related data that can shape our assessment of human illness....Through the lens of the digital phenotype, an individual's interaction with digital technologies affects the full spectrum of human disease from diagnosis, to treatment, to chronic disease management."[369]

There are many opportunities this approach brings to health: consider forecasting and tracking epidemics, which Dr. Brownstein has done by building public health surveillance tools like HealthMap. HealthMap brings together online news stories, blog posts, and social data to forecast disease outbreaks and real-time surveillance of emerging public health trends. Digital phenotyping can also help to improve clinical trials for new therapies, better manage chronic disease, harness self-tracking data for research, and, enable patients to more effectively focus on individual health goals.[370]

But take note: lots of this information isn't specifically "healthcare" data and, as such, isn't covered by HIPAA. Generally, all personal data collected on an individual by a HIPAA covered entity (such as a health care provider or health insurer) is considered to be PHI and therefore covered by HIPAA.[371]

Still, aggregating person-generated data from outside of the healthcare system is useful for healthcare purposes. Patients, though, have been largely unaware of the data that "leaks" out of their daily life-flows.[372]

Data, data everywhere: the privacy challenge

"Data collected in doctors' offices are afforded one type of protection, but we do not have in place the legal frameworks that offer protections to similar data gathered from our smartphones, web searches, and digital devices," wrote Gina Neff and Dawn Nafus in their book, *Self-Tracking*.[373]

As more people leave more digital footprints online every day, there are opportunities for both positive data mining – as the previous chapter described – and not-so-sanguine applications. Consider the social network Facebook, which is well-utilized as a convening platform for patients managing chronic disease.[374] On the upside, there is a growing evidence base that patient social networks can boost peoples' knowledge, competence, and health outcomes. A group of surgeons found that creating a Facebook support group for liver transplant patients boosted positive impacts on patient care, greater engagement and satisfaction.[375]

On the public health front, *ProPublica* organized a Facebook group with over one thousand members to share stories, swap advice and engage in dialogue on patient harm and medical errors. This has evolved into an important resource for public health researchers, providers, and journalists looking into the ongoing challenge of patient harm.[376]

But, "data mining and profiling methods, in combining diverse data sets on people, can begin to reveal very detailed and sensitive information about them in ways these individuals may not have anticipated when they granted consent to the use of their data."[377] It is likely that many people who upload and share their personal health information are not aware of the extent to which their data might be shared with third parties not identified in the privacy policy they signed to gain access to the social network or app, or that their data might be used in ways not disclosed in the app or social network's privacy policy.

A vivid example of this involved a young woman and the retailer Target. A clever statistician at the company figured out how to mine retail receipts for purchased items like supplements (calcium, magnesium and zinc), nausea meds and a list of about 25 products that, together, informed a pregnancy-predictability statistical model.

"We knew that if we could identify them [the prospective mothers] in their second trimester, there's a good chance we could capture them for years," the statistician told Charles Duhigg, the *New York Times* reporter who detailed this story. "As soon as we get them buying diapers from us, they're going to start buying everything else too," the Target employee said.

The retailer targeted mailings to these women identified in the model. One day, a man walked into a Target store and asked to see the manager, Duhigg reported, the man presenting a pile of coupons sent to his daughter. "My daughter got this in the mail! She's still in high school, and you're sending her coupons for baby clothes and cribs? Are you trying to encourage her to get pregnant?" Duhigg quoted.

The upshot: as it turned out, the man's daughter was indeed already pregnant, and he did not know.[378]

His daughter's digital footprints, that she unwittingly left through retail receipts and social media posts, were data points that the Target mathematician could cleverly lasso into a predictive algorithm.

The apps conundrum – a "concerned embrace" of technology

People use their mobile phones like Swiss Army knives, Susannah Fox told me many years ago as she was studying the growing role of mobile for health at the Pew Research Group.

Given the nature of digital dust thrown off by peoples' use of mobile for daily living, we must consider consumers' "concerned embrace" of technology as people weigh security and privacy risks in the context of their demand for convenience.[379]

Scientific American published an article in the Health section titled, "For Sale: Your Medical Records." The essay explained the growing and profitable business for companies that collect, analyze, and package consumers' personal information and sell it as a commodity without peoples' knowledge. This was first highlighted in mass media

SOURCES OF YOUR DATA

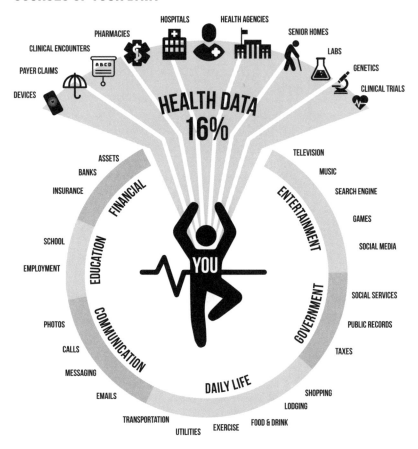

Source: Adapted from Sources of Your Data, GoInvo and Juhan Sonin, February 2019

by *60 Minutes* in March 2014 in a story titled, "The Data Brokers." [380]

Most consumers are unaware what HIPAA covers, and knowing about these data flows would no doubt surprise many people. Latanya Sweeney's team at the Data Privacy Lab at Harvard University identified the flows of personal information that fell outside of HIPAA privacy protections. The team began this work in 2010, which was a time when consumers got comfortable using the Internet to conduct various tasks: paying bills online, downloading music, and seeking health information on medical websites. While 61 percent of Americans sought such health information online, only 10 percent of U.S. doctors used a fully functional electronic health record (EHR) system at the time.[381]

This changed with the implementation of the HITECH Act. Data held in the EHR by a hospital, clinic, or physician, is covered by the HIPAA Privacy and Security Rules.

By 2019, there were over 318,000 digital health apps available in app stores worldwide. Mental health is the largest focus for disease-specific mobile apps, with tools to help people dealing with autism, depression, and anxiety, among other issues. While most apps have fewer than 5,000 downloads, the most popular apps have been downloaded by millions of users.[382]

Each click onto a mobile app or Internet health search creates a bit of digital dust which can flow outside of HIPAA's scope. The Harvard Data Privacy Project studied several dozen popular health and fitness apps and concluded that there were privacy risks for users which the apps' privacy policies did not describe. The Project also noted that these apps were popular because they offer benefits, convenience, and often free access using them. Thus, consumers should not assume their "health" and "sensitive" data — such as weight, mood, or disease status — is private in a mobile app environment, the Privacy Rights Clearinghouse recommended.[383]

HIPAA is one piece in a patchwork quilt of privacy trying to protect Americans.

HIPAA – what it does and doesn't cover

HIPAA was signed into law by President Clinton in 1996. After signing the legislation, President Clinton said, "For the first time, this Act will ensure the portability of health benefits when workers change or lose their jobs," and, "It provides for the development of: (1) national standards for the electronic submission of health insurance claims that will reduce paperwork, administrative costs, and burdens for doctors and hospitals; and (2) privacy protection recommendations for health information generally, and, in the absence of additional legislation, regulations for privacy of health care claims information." [384]

The second part of President Clinton's statement focused on the "Accountability" part of HIPAA, meant to protect health data availability, confidentiality, and integrity. The drafters of the law understood that doctors and hospitals had begun to transfer patients' medical records to electronic forms, and so incorporated provisions to protect individually identifiable health information to ensure privacy.

HIPAA requires so-called covered entities and business associates to ensure the privacy and security of personally-identifiable health related data. Covered entities are most health care providers (those who perform "covered transactions" – usually health insurance payment-related transactions - for which HHS has adopted standards), health plans (health insurance companies, HMOs, company health plans, government programs that pay for health care like Medicare, Medicare, the military and Veterans Health programs), and health care clearinghouses. Specific roles underneath these categories include doctors, clinics, psychologists, dentists, chiropractors, nursing homes, and pharmacies.

Who's not included on this list? Wearable technology companies and mobile health app developers. Data that is collected by consumers via wearable devices, apps, and other digital tech is HIPAA-covered only when it is in the possession of the HIPAA-covered entity (e.g., hospitals, doctors, and pharmacies).[385]

Mending the holes in Americans' privacy patchwork quilt

Where Europeans benefit from a "blanket" of privacy protection in the Global Data Privacy Regulation (GDPR), Americans are under a regulatory patchwork quilt.[386]

In the U.S., there are several laws outside of HIPAA that touch on Americans' privacy including:

- The Children's Online Privacy Protection Act (COPPA), which applies to websites and online services collecting information on children under 13 years of age
- The FTC Act, addressing companies' protection of consumers' personal information, separate from HIPAA
- Genetic Information and Nondiscrimination Act (GINA), protecting people against discrimination based on their genetic information in health coverage and employment, among other regulations that deal with some aspect of health privacy
- SAMHSA Part 2 rules, which protect substance abuse treatment data in the hands of federally supported substance abuse treatment programs.

Beyond wearable tech for health, apps, and FDA-cleared remote health monitoring devices, there are other sources never imagined by the folks who drafted the HIPAA language in 1996. Consider the connected car as a health data source (discussed in the *Digital Health* chapter), morphing into a potential health data leakage channel. In the growing Internet of Healthy Things, information flows go well beyond those conceived by the framers of HIPAA.

As new automobiles come onto the market, they are connected to the Internet. In 2017, the volume of new cars added to cellular networks exceeded the number of new cellphone accounts. [387] Why is this important? Because car companies are positioning to sell drivers' data to companies that deal in consumer information.[388]

Most consumers are unaware of the connected car's ability to store personal identified information. Interestingly, privacy and cybersecurity were the biggest business and legal issues that auto industry executives identified in the connected car era in a survey conducted by the law firm, Foley and Lardner LLP. Auto industry thought leaders ranked privacy and cybersecurity well above safety concerns, capabilities of the technology, and cost. [389]

To help mitigate and risk-manage the emerging challenge of connected cars and cyber-hacking, the Automotive Information Sharing and Analysis Center (ISAC) was formed to prevent, respond to, and help recover from cyber-threats to connected cars.[390] Auto-ISAC was formed in 2015 by the Auto Alliance, a global association of automakers, to share and analyze intelligence about cybersecurity risks to cars. The A-ISAC is one of several ISACs representing other industry sectors, all formed in response to President Obama's policy directive on Critical Infrastructure Security and Resilience launched in 2013. The directive was issued to strengthen the U.S. infrastructure to withstand and recover from hazards – including cyber-threats.[391]

A Government Accountability Office report studied the privacy policies of sixteen automakers who manufactured connected cars. The GAO found that none of the connected carmakers offered clearly-written privacy policies, nor did the companies identify data sharing and use practices. GAO recommended that the National Highway Traffic Safety Administration define and communicate its roles and responsibilities for privacy of data generated by and collected from vehicles.[392]

"Your driving behavior, location, has monetary value, not unlike your search activity, recognized Roger Lanctot, an expert on connected autos with Strategy Analytics.[393] Most drivers in the U.S. switching on Bluetooth in their automobiles are largely unaware of what aspects of their health information are protected, and which are not.

While most western countries have adopted over-arching data protection for their citizens, the United States has not. Americans are global outliers when it comes to (weaker) data privacy protection.

The U.S., "home to some of the most advanced, and largest, technology and data companies in the world, continues to lumber forward with a patchwork of sector-specific laws and regulations that fail to adequately protect data," Nuala O'Connor, President and CEP of the Center for Democracy and Technology, asserted in a Council on Foreign Relations report.[394] "It is past time for Congress to create a single legislative data-protection mandate to protect individuals' privacy and reconcile the differences between state and federal requirements," she recommended. Doing so would bring the U.S. in line with emerging data-protection norms, O'Connor noted – especially important for bolstering Americans' health data privacy protection and personal empowerment.

Learning from Hugo and Joe

Hugo Campus is alive and well, powered by both an indomitable creative spirit and an implanted cardiac defibrillator (ICD) which he's had since 2007. Hugo was diagnosed with hypertrophic cardiomyopathy, a condition where the heart muscle becomes abnormally thick, making it harder for the heart to pump blood. This can result in life-threatening abnormal heart rhythm and sudden death.

"It's the same disease that causes 17-year-olds to suddenly drop dead on the soccer field," Amy Standen wrote in her profile on Hugo for NPR.[395]

As an engaged patient, Hugo wanted access to the data that was being collected by the ICD device. In 2012, he approached Medtronic, the manufacturer of the device, about accessing that data. The company was resistant in giving Hugo the information, explaining to Standen, "You want to do it in a way that makes sense for the patient, that they can interpret correctly, so they don't generate a lot of angst and difficulty for the physician or anyone else."

Hugo's response was, "Whether I can make sense of it or not, it's another problem. I should be allowed at least to have a chance to look at this data and see if I can make sense of it."

Just about a year later, the CEO of Medtronic tweeted the following: "Using Runtastic to track progress with running; find it motivating & pushes me to improve. Here is my morning run," coupled with an image of the data from the run.[396]

Hugo, active on social media, tweeted in response, "@MedtronicCEO Thumbs up on using #mHealth apps to track progress. Thumbs down for not giving same access to patients with your devices #FAIL."

Soon after that tweet-exchange, Medtronic contacted Hugo to work out a way for his clinicians at Stanford Hospital & Clinics to share the data with him. But the manual process proved convoluted and onerous on the clinic and was soon abandoned.

Data tracked by a medical device company like Medtronic is largely considered to fall outside of HIPAA law. Strictly in terms of the law, a medical device company is not compelled to share patient-generated data.

Hugo's story highlights the importance of a patient's tenacity in seeking their data, and the growing role that social media and online patient social networks can play in solidifying patient power, amplifying individual patient voices.

"For Campos, data ownership was not about an obscure legal theory. The data was the stuff of his body, and he wanted it back."[397]

Vice President Joe Biden echoed Hugo's demand for his patient data at a meeting of the Cancer Moonshot in August 2017. Judith Faulkner, CEO of Epic, a market leader in electronic health records systems, asked Biden, "Why do you want your medical records? They're a thousand pages of which you understand 10."

The Vice President responded, "None of your business."[398]

What if... America reduced health disparities, increased health equity, and our ZIP codes didn't determine our health outcomes and life expectancy?

Chapter 7

ZIP CODES, GENTETIC CODES, FOOD AND HEALTH

ZIP codes and genetic codes: place matters for health

There's a 15 year difference in the life expectancy between the richest and poorest Americans.[399]

That gap is largely attributable to geography. *Place matters* for a person's health.

Using the shiniest, newest digital health technologies won't, in and of themselves, mitigate the risk factors that shape our health before and at birth, during childhood, and throughout life.

The social determinants of health (SDoHs) are the conditions in which people are born, grow, work, live, and age.[400] Think: economic stability, income, and socioeconomic status; employment and working conditions; education; neighborhood, housing, physical environment, clean air and water; food; community and social support; and, access to healthcare services.

One-half of the deaths in the U.S. in 1990 resulted from some combination of external factors: tobacco use, diet and activity patterns, alcohol, microbial agents, toxic agents, firearms, sexual behavior, motor vehicles, and illicit use of drugs.[401] McGinnis and Foege published this finding in an influential 1993 *JAMA* essay, among the earliest quantitative studies into the social determinants of health. "The most important implications of this assessment of the actual causes of death in the United States are found in the way the nation allocates its social resources," the authors wrote.

When McGinnis and Foege asserted that, health care costs in the U.S. reached $900 billion. "The preponderance of this expenditure," they calculated, "will be devoted to treatment of conditions ultimately recorded on death certificates as the nation's leading killers. Only a small fraction will go to control of many of the factors" that imposed a substantial public health burden."

Nearly twenty years before McGinnis and Foege identified social determinants' influence on Americans' health, Thomas McKeown was doing the same for people living in England. McKeown wrote about *The Role of Medicine: Dream, Mirage or Nemesis?* in 1976, citing the positive health influence that nutrition, environment, and access to vaccines had on increasing longevity in Great Britain.[402]

"The requirements for health can be stated simply," McKeown wrote. "Those fortunate enough to be born free of significant congenital disease or disability will remain well if three basic needs are met: they must be adequately fed; they must be protected from a wide range of hazards in the environment; and they must not depart radically from the pattern of personal behaviour under which man evolved, for example by smoking, overeating, or sedentary living."

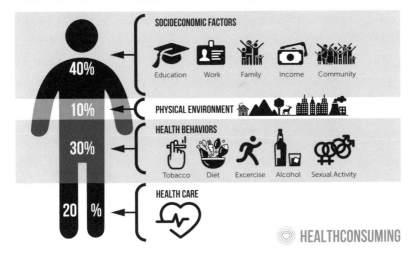

THE SOCIAL DETERMINANTS OF HEALTH:
HEALTH MADE BY MANY FACTORS BEYOND HEALTH CARE

Source: Schroeder SA.
We Can Do Better -
Improving the Health of
the American People.
NEJM 357.1221-8, 2007

The social determinants of health

"There are places where you pay a price in the loss of life because of your address," Dr. Anthony Iton figured out as health director for Alameda County in 2008. Analyzing death certificate data by age, race, ethnicity, and neighborhood, Iton's team was among the first to find life expectancy differences in the same city that were as wide as 20 years apart.[403]

Dr. Iton was, arguably, the first person to coin that our ZIP code is more important than our genetic code. Dr. Iton's work determined that a person's geographic "place" defined their access to clean water, good education, walkable streets, green spaces, and nutritious food.

The social determinants of health have quantifiable and lifelong health impacts for people.

Socioeconomic status: Income, education, and occupation make up a person's socioeconomic status (SES). There is a strong statistical relationship between a person's socioeconomic status and their health. The bottom-line on SES and health in the United States: wealthy people tend to be healthier than people of poorer status.[404] SES is linked to a broad range of health problems from low birthweight at the beginning of life;[405] arthritis, cancer, diabetes, hypertension as people age;[406] and ultimately, higher mortality in adulthood.[407] Low-birth weight is a measure of health at the "starting gate" of life as a risk factor for infant mortality and a marker for child morbidity among infants who survive. In the U.S., disparities in health at birth are wider than in Australia, Canada, and the United Kingdom.[408] The three countries' more generous social support and health care system designs play buffering roles.

Education: Education is a key component of SES. When policymakers debate the benefits of increasing access to education, they rarely account for improvements in population health.[409] Education lays the foundation for future job opportunities and earning potential. Education also bolsters literacy and life skills that allow people to more readily access information and resources to promote health.[410] The health gaps between better educated and less educated men and women have widened over time. When race and education are combined, these health disparities are even wider.[411]

Health system literacy: Beyond the consideration of general education, it must be noted that health literacy in America is multi-layered. Being an engaged health consumer in the U.S. requires many competencies: general healthcare literacy (e.g., understanding how to take a prescribed medicine or instructions for continuing physical therapy at home), health plan literacy (e.g., understanding how to navigate one's health insurance), financial literacy (e.g., why and how to invest in a health savings account or the definition of "coinsurance"), digital literacy (e.g., how to access a health insurance marketplace and sign up for insurance, or how to search for credible medical advice online), and privacy rights literacy (e.g., how to interpret privacy policies for a mobile app or what HIPAA covers). At least one in four consumers had a low understanding of the U.S. health system in 2018: Accenture calculated a savings of $3.4 billion a year just for administrative expenses if all consumers understood how to navigate U.S. health care.[412]

Job insecurity and unemployment: The feeling that one could lose their job, job-insecurity, is a health risk factor impacting mental and physical health.[413] Studies show that the fear of job loss among a blue collar workforce is a risk for workers' physical decline.[414, 415] The negative impacts of losing a job and being unemployed go beyond the effects on income and damage people's overall well-being regardless of age, gender, level of education, or ethnicity.[416]

Social connection and loneliness: Older people who are lonely have a higher risk of death as well as being more challenged in performing everyday tasks.[417] People who are socially isolated or lonely also have a much greater risk of developing dementia,[418] a higher risk for cardiovascular disease,[419] and are four times more likely to be re-hospitalized within a year of being discharged from the hospital.[420] Isolation may also cause changes in the body such as inflammation and poor immune functioning, leading to premature death.[421]

Social isolation costs Medicare $6.7 billion annually, from spending on avoidable hospitalization and nursing home care. That amounts to an additional $134 per Medicare enrollee, comparable to an additional $163 per member for high blood pressure and $117 per enrollee for arthritis.[422]

Food security: Food insecurity is defined as lacking consistent access to enough food for active, healthy living. About 12 percent of U.S. households were food insecure in 2017, still above the pre-Recession level of 11.1 percent.[423] Food insecurity is a risk for increased prevalence of illness and poor chronic disease management.[424] Food insecure households spend 45 percent more on medical care than people in food-secure homes. People with food insecurity are 50 percent more likely to have diabetes and 60 percent more likely to have congestive heart failure or experience a heart attack;[425] visit the emergency room more frequently;[426] and, have higher rates of hospital admissions and longer stays in the hospital.[427] Food insecurity has also been linked to depression, especially acute among children growing up in low-income homes.[428, 429] Food security is a function of place, income and culture, where people might be able to afford healthy food but can benefit from learning more about nutrition and how to cook healthy meals with locally available ingredients.

Transportation: Transportation impacts peoples' health in several ways. People who lack access to transportation are more likely to delay care, miss appointments with doctors and clinics, and miss or delay medication use.[430] One in four lower-income patients have missed or rescheduled appointments due to lack of transportation, which costs U.S. health providers as much as $150 billion annually.[431] The second transportation-health impact is that active transportation – walking, bicycling, and public transit – gets people moving and playing in neighborhoods. However, in lower-income communities, residents often lack safe and convenient access to get to work, school, healthy food shopping, and healthcare appointments.[432]

Smoking: More than ten times as many U.S. citizens have died prematurely from cigarette smoking than have died in all the wars fought by the U.S. Smoking increases risk for death from all causes

POOR AIR QUALITY CUTS LIFE EXPECTANCY MORE THAN SMOKING, ALCOHOL AND DRUG USE, UNSAFE WATER, AND HIV/AIDS

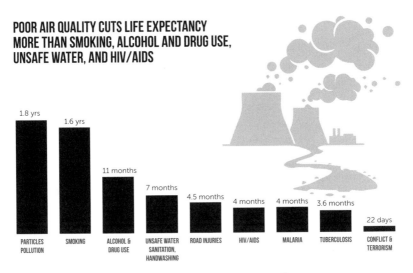

PARTICLES POLLUTION	SMOKING	ALCOHOL & DRUG USE	UNSAFE WATER SANITATION, HANDWASHING	ROAD INJURIES	HIV/AIDS	MALARIA	TUBERCULOSIS	CONFLICT & TERRORISM
1.8 yrs	1.6 yrs	11 months	7 months	4.5 months	4 months	4 months	3.6 months	22 days

Source: Air Quality Life Index, EPIC, University of Chicago, November 2018

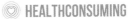

HEALTHCONSUMING

in men and women: for coronary heart disease, stroke, and for cancers throughout the body. If no one smoked, one in every three cancer deaths in the U.S. would not happen.[433]

Clean air: Particulate air pollution cuts the average person's life span by 2 years.[434] The health impact of particulate pollution is comparable to that of smoking. While the U.S. has made progress on improving air quality, with 85 percent of the U.S. population breathing clean air, some counties have particulate concentrations below the World Health Organization guidelines: for example, in California, where people in Los Angeles would live about six months longer if WHO recommendations were met; and, in Arizona, Illinois, Indiana and Ohio, with higher-than-optimal levels of particulate pollution. Most pollution-related deaths occur in low-income and middle-income places. Children face the highest risks because small exposures to chemicals in early childhood can result in lifelong disease, disability, premature death, and reduced learning and earning potentials.[435] The U.S. made significant improvements in air quality between 1990 and 2010. However, particulate matter and ozone continue to threaten public health, with over 58,000 deaths a year attributable to air pollution.[436]

Clean water: Some 63 million people in the U.S. (about one in five) were exposed to potentially unsafe water between 2007 and 2017, according to water quality and monitoring violations from the from the Environmental Protection Agency.[437] The U.S. scored a grade of "D" from the American Society of Civil Engineers for the quality of the nation's drinking water systems based on an evaluation of their safety, condition, and capacity. No state scored higher than a "C+."[438] The health impacts of unsafe water range from diarrhea and nausea to skin rashes, cancer, reproductive problems, and developmental delays after drinking water for a long period of time.[439]

Climate change: "Impacts from climate change on extreme weather and climate-related events, air quality, and the transmission of disease through insects and pests, food, and water increasingly threaten the health and well-being of the American people, particularly populations that are already vulnerable," the fourth national climate assessment report noted in 2018. The report forecasted growing air quality and health risks due to wildfire and ground-level ozone pollution, heat-related deaths, and greater exposure to waterborne and foodborne diseases that will threaten food and water safety along with raising the risk of respiratory and allergic illnesses. The report emphasized that populations including older adults, children, low-income communities, and some communities of color are often disproportionately affected by, and less resilient to, the health impacts of climate change.[440]

Healthy housing: Public health advocates link health outcomes like asthma, lead poisoning, and unintentional injuries, with home health hazards.[441] The National Center for

Healthy Housing offers an eight-point framework for healthy homes with the principles of building and keeping homes that are dry, clean, pest-free, safe, contaminant-free, ventilated, maintained, and thermally-controlled. Damp houses are a breeding-ground for mites, rodents and mold, all risk factors for asthma. Most injuries among children occur at home including falls, burns, and poisonings. Chemical exposures to asbestos, radon gas, carbon monoxide, and secondhand tobacco smoke are greater indoors than outdoors. Older homes are at-risk for deteriorated lead-based paint; lead is highly toxic and can cause damage to the brain, the kidneys, nervous system and blood, especially in young children. While lead-based paint was banned in in the U.S. in 1978, over 24 million aging homes still have deteriorated lead paint.[442]

Access to healthcare services: Medical care alone is estimated to account for only 10 to 20 percent of the modifiable contributors to health outcomes.[443] But lack of access to medical services can be a barrier to good health. Access to health care is the timely use of personal health services to achieve the best possible health outcomes, the National Academies of Sciences, Engineering and Medicine defined in 1993.[444] Barriers to healthcare include poor access to transportation, institutional prejudice, lack of availability of services, professional shortage areas, lack of health insurance coverage, the high cost of care, and lack of culturally competent care (e.g., language). These barriers can result in delays in receiving appropriate care, unmet health needs, preventable hospitalizations, and financial burdens (often resulting in personal bankruptcy, discussed in *The Patient Is the Payor*).

But for mainstream consumers to benefit from digital health innovations, there's an underpinning that's key to making that happen: connectivity and broadband.

Broadband connectivity is a social determinant of health

Since the emergence of America Online, CompuServe and Prodigy, online listservs and patient groups have supported peoples' health. Today, without online access, people can't apply to jobs (which support financial security), find information on essential social services, shop for health insurance, access educational opportunities, or stay connected on social networks that can be a literal lifeline for people who may feel a taboo about face-to-face encounters with medical professionals (say, mental health providers).

Twenty years ago, when I co-wrote the paper *Health e-People* with Institute for the Future colleagues, we identified a digital divide in America.[445] This was particularly acute between whites compared with African-American and Hispanic people. The digital divide of have's and have not's has, notably, been between healthy people and people managing more than one chronic condition; and, people in rural areas, who can lack access to healthcare providers, specialists, and mental health services.

Availability of high-quality broadband is necessary to address the digital healthcare divide. The U.S. Department of Agriculture projected the need for high-quality household broadband service will likely increase if patients are to avail themselves of new telehealth and digital health services, especially in rural and poor areas where low quality broadband Internet service tends to be more common.[446] People who live in rural areas also lag behind urban residents when paying medical bills online, emailing with healthcare providers, and monitoring health online by a factor of two to one, urban vs. rural patients.

Without broadband connectivity, the nation's residents can't fully benefit from the promise of digital health technology. One key ingredient missing from digital health Nirvana is the deployment of broadband connectivity in every community in America – not to the proverbial "last mile," but to the last person.

Even with the presence of broadband, the cost of data plans can be prohibitive to lower-income people – many dealing with chronic health conditions. Broadband is now a social determinant of health.[447] The FCC recognized that, "health care is being transformed by the availability and accessibility of broadband-enabled services and technologies and the development of life-saving wireless medical devices."[448] Without connectivity to the internet, people in under-served communities cannot uniformly receive evidence-based, timely, appropriate healthcare or participate in research trials.[449]

Social determinants impact healthcare spending

A decade after Dr. Iton published the public health research on Alameda County, the Blue Cross Blue Shield Association asked, "Why are some communities healthier than others?" Working with Moody's Analytics, BCBSA mined the health records of 40 million members of insurance plans and found that five conditions nationally were responsible for a huge chronic disease burden in the U.S.: depression, hypertension, diabetes, high cholesterol, and substances use disorders.[450] Socioeconomic and behavioral factors were found to be significantly more powerful influencers on these conditions' outcomes compared with receiving medical services.

High cholesterol, coronary artery disease, hypertension, COPD and diabetes are highly related to places where smoking and obesity are more prevalent, and where people have lower levels of physical activity.

Smoking, obesity and sedentary lifestyles are obvious behaviors that negatively impact health. But there are other factors that can exacerbate medical conditions. Consider a person with diabetes and her lens on daily living. In addition to the visible factors of smoking, obesity and less physical activity, Gallup and Sharecare's Well-Being Index found that communities with higher prevalence of diabetes had lower percentages of people who felt proud of their community. Fewer residents in high-diabetes prevalence communities also felt that they were thriving.[451]

These conditions are also amenable to people making lifestyle changes and accessing relevant social services that can support people in self-care – consuming nutritious food, being more physically active, not smoking or quitting tobacco, reaching out for social opportunities, and accessing health care services when needed without delay.

Healthcare spending can be reduced when people are connected to social services that address barriers to the social determinants of health, like secure housing, medical transportation, nutritional food programs, utility assistance, social communities, and on-ramps to employment.[452]

Ranking social spending the U.S.

Noting the predominance of acute care in England's NHS budget, McKeown wrote in his 1976 book, "What is needed is an adjustment in the balance of interest and resources between the three main areas of service...the personal and non-personal influences which are the major determinants of health: to food and the environment, which will be mainly in the hands of specialists, and to personal behaviour, which should be the concern of every practicing doctor. These interests should no longer be peripheral to the medical role."[453]

Compared with other wealthy nations, the U.S. allocates a markedly smaller proportion of gross domestic product on social spending relative to health care.

The chart compares the U.S. to other OECD countries' rate of life expectancy at birth versus national health spending as a percentage of GDP, and then the percent of GDP allocated to social spending as a multiple of healthcare spending.

In the U.S., only about 10 percent more of GDP is spent on social care, compared with the high of 2.7 times in France, 2.5 times in Sweden, and 2.4 times in Norway – all with greater life expectancy outcomes.

HEALTHCARE SPENDING AND LIFE EXPECTANCY AT BIRTH SELECTED OECD COUNTRIES

	LIFE EXPECTANCY AT BIRTH, 2016	HEALTHCARE SPENDING % OF GDP, 2017	% OF GDP ALLOCATED TO SOCIAL SPENDING AS MULTIPLE OF % OF GDP FOR HEALTHCARE
France	82.4	11.5%	2.7x
Sweden	82.4	10.9%	2.5x
Switzerland	83.7	12.3%	1.6x
Germany	81.1	11.3%	2.3x
Netherlands	81.5	10.1%	2.2x
U.S.	78.6	17.2%	1.1x
Norway	82.5	10.4%	2.4x
U.K.	81.2	9.7%	2.2x
New Zealand	81.7	9.0%	2.1x
Canada	81.9	10.4%	1.7x
Australia	82.5	9.1%	2.1x

Source: OECD Health Statistics, 2018; OECD Health at a Glance, 2017   HEALTHCONSUMING

Residents in every one of these countries also benefit from coverage through some form of universal health care insurance. The design of these insurance plans varies from country to country, but all – except for the United States – ensure health services for every person in the nation.

Health where we live, work, play, pray and learn

The American College of Physicians published a position paper on addressing social determinants to improve patient care and health equity. In the document, this group of 154,000 doctors, the largest medical society in the world, called social determinants, "an important component of the physician's role as an advocate for patients and a steward of medical care."[454]

Our communities are our local health ecosystems. Centuries-worth of evidence, from Hippocrates in Athens, Greece to Geisinger Medical Center in Danville, PA, shows us that how we live, the daily choices we make or are constrained from making, and the built and natural environments we live in shape our health well beyond the local doctor and hospital do.

What if...people in America were Health Citizens, where the government ensured health care as a social and civil right, health informed public policy, and people owned and controlled their health data? What if home was our health hub?

Chapter 8

BECOMING HEALTH CITIZENS

Most Americans like the idea of healthcare as a national right

Healthcare was the top issue driving the 2018 U.S. midterm elections. Nearly one-half of the ads aired for U.S. Senate races for Democrats were about health care versus 24 percent for Republicans.

While the "caravan" and Supreme Court appointments garnered national headlines, health care did not. But the issue drove voters to the polls, prompting the Wesleyan Media Project to conclude, "It's official: The 2018 midterms are about health care."[455]

What motivated these healthcare voters was their collective concern about healthcare costs and access to care.

The vast majority of Americans support affordable health care as a right across political party lines: 99 percent of Democrats, 82 percent of Republicans, and 92 percent of Independents. In a Commonwealth

Fund poll, support for affordable care as a right garnered nearly all people, regardless of race or ethnicity. The same held for insurance status, whether the consumer was commercially insured by an employer or enrolled in Medicaid, Medicare, through a health insurance marketplace, or uninsured.[456]

Weeks before the 2018 mid-terms, more than 50 percent of Republicans expressed support for a Medicare for All plan in a Reuters poll.[457] This represented a shift that Sarah Kliff uncovered in 2017 after visiting Kentucky and meeting with registered Republicans in the state who enrolled in Obamacare, had voted for Donald Trump for President, and began to understand what eroding or repealing the Affordable Care Act could mean for them in terms of losing their coverage, and ultimately health and financial security.[458]

In November 2018, during the week of the mid-term elections, half of Americans said it was a major concern that they would not have enough money to pay for medical care, and 61 percent worried that their health plan would charge higher premiums. The issue of pre-existing conditions also posed major concerns for consumers, four in ten of whom said they worried about a loved one being denied health coverage.[459]

While it's no surprise that lower-income Americans were highly concerned about paying higher premiums, most people earning over $75,000 a year were also very worried about covering the costs of health insurance. This was also equally true for people whether enrolled in Medicare, Medicaid, or covered by private insurance.

By late 2018, seven in ten Americans had a negative view of the U.S. health care system.[460]   Ultimately, Gallup found that most Americans favored the government ensuring healthcare for all.

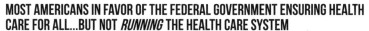

MOST AMERICANS IN FAVOR OF THE FEDERAL GOVERNMENT ENSURING HEALTH CARE FOR ALL...BUT NOT *RUNNING* THE HEALTH CARE SYSTEM

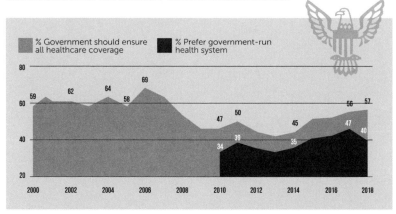

Source: Gallup, Government Favored to Ensure Healthcare, but Not Deliver It, December 3, 2018

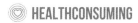 HEALTHCONSUMING

It's not only patients who believe in universal healthcare for fellow Americans; it's most doctors, too. The American Medical Association came out in January 2017 with a statement in the journal *JAMA* titled, "Health Care in the United States: A Right or a Privilege."[461]

"I hope that all physicians, including those who are members of Congress, other health care professionals, and professional societies would speak with a single voice and say that health care is a basic right for every person, and not a privilege to be available and affordable only for a majority," Dr. Bauchner of the AMA urged his fellow doctors. "The solution for how to achieve health care coverage for all may be uniquely American, but it is an exceedingly important and worthy goal, emblematic of a fair and just society."

In that statement, Dr. Bauchner channeled elements of the Hippocratic Oath from a modern version attributed to Louis Lasagna, Academic Dean of the School of Medicine at Tufts

University. Updated in 1964, the modernized Oath read in part: "I will prevent disease whenever I can, for prevention is preferable to cure. I will remember that I remain a member of society, with special obligations to all my fellow human beings."[462]

Speaking Greek for health

The Hippocratic Oath was composed in Ancient Greece, the birthplace of democracy, by that ancient Greek Hippocrates in the collection of medical works known as *The Corpus*, considered one of the first medical textbooks.[463] Dating back to the 5th century BC, the work rocked the Greek Classic period's medical world by pointing to social, physical, and nutritional influences on health and wellbeing, breaking traditional medicine away from prevailing superstitious and magical therapeutic teachings.

Specifically, the discussion of "diatetica" or "diatia" in the book was broader than "diet" as contemporary western medicine teaches. The Greeks' concept for diet went beyond food, recognizing the health-promoting roles of sleep, exercise, healthy living (such as moderate wine consumption[464]), and finally "place," which Hippocrates *et.al.* covered in the *Air, Waters, Places* section of the *Corpus*. This guided Greece's traveling physicians to understand patients' exposure to the three physical elements to anticipate what diseases they were likely to encounter when setting up practice in new, unfamiliar towns.[465]

The Hippocratic clinicians classified disease into two categories: endemic, which were conditions usually present in populations; and epidemic, which occurred only at certain times in certain people. In *Air, Water and Places*, Team Hippocrates discussed key factors in "endemicity," such as climate, soil quality, nutrition, lifestyle and housing – that is, in today's parlance, medical geography. "Those [cities] facing the rising sun are naturally more healthy than those facing north and those facing south, even though the distance between them be only a single stadium," the work asserted.[466] Hippocrates advised doctors to inquire into patients' dwellings, proximity to the sea, exposure to the wind, and quality of water accessible to peoples' homes.

Consider Flint, Michigan's public health challenge two thousand years after Hippocrates' teachings. In the 21st century, the Hippocratic lessons equate to recognizing that our ZIP code is at least as important as our genetic code. Living in Flint was a health risk for thousands of people exposed to a tainted water supply, putting the town's children at-risk for developmental delays[467] and adults with compromised gut issues, heart disease,[468] and emotional distress.[469]

Doctors were also taught through Hippocratic texts to consider the social and political status of their patients, which shaped lifestyles and, ultimately health.[470] Hippocratic writings refer to the "health of the polis."

"The institution of democracy and the state's responsibility for justice and education...reflected a supportive social environment for health and the promotion of healthy attitudes and behaviors," Yannis Tountas wrote explaining the roots of health promotion and education in Greek philosophy.[471]

From Hippocrates to Christakis: health is social

TIME magazine identified the most influential Greek-American of 2009 as Nicholas Christakis.[472] Christakis's research realized that our individual health is connected to the health of people in our social networks: those in our immediate circles, as well as networks of people in our friends' circles of social influence.[473]

Simply put, social relationships – in terms of both quantity and quality - affect health behaviors, physical health, mental health, and mortality risks.

"People are interconnected, and so their health is interconnected," Christakis co-wrote with his colleague Kirsten Smith in an essay on social networks and health.[474] Earlier work by Cassel, Cobb, and Berkman demonstrated that social networks could affect mortality, learning that death in one person can be associated with similar outcomes in other people to whom that person is tied – illustrating the non-biological transmission of illness.[475] Older people who were socially isolated were 50 percent more likely to die than people who were well-connected.[476]

"Loneliness is an epidemic in plain sight. We treat it as an unavoidable part of aging," Dr. Sachin Jain, CEO of CareMore, has observed.[477]

People are connected for health in obesity, smoking, binge drinking, and other lifestyle behaviors that directly impact health. Furthermore, social relationships are associated with physical health markers like blood pressure and C-reactive protein. Social isolation has also been found to increase the risk of inflammation by the same magnitude as physical inactivity in adolescence.[478]

"Our connections do not end with the people we know. Beyond our own social horizons, friends of friends of friends can start chain reactions that eventually reach us, like waves from distant lands that wash up on our shores," Christakis and co-author James Fowler explained in their book, Connected.[479]

Loneliness is contagious. In his study Alone in the Crowd, Dr. John Cacioppo collaborated with Fowler and Christakis to mine the landmark Framingham Heart Study and found that the spread of loneliness is stronger than the spread of perceived social connections.[480] "People on the edge of the network spread their loneliness to others and then cut their ties," the trio wrote, finding, "an extraordinary pattern of contagion...[leading[people to be moved to the edge of the social network when they become lonely...on the periphery people have fewer friends, yet their loneliness leads them to losing the few ties they have left." They compared this process to that of the loose ends of a crocheted sweater that, with the pull of one thread, can unravel the entire garment. That is the counter-metaphor for a healthy, tightly-woven social fabric.

Senator Tip O'Neill's old saw that "all politics is local" inspired the mantra that, "all healthcare is local." But healthcare's not just local anymore. It's social.[481]

The American epidemic of deaths of despair

In addition to social connection, education is one of the most impactful social determinants for health, discussed in the *ZIP Codes* chapter. The lack of education has been found to be just as deadly as a pack of cigarettes smoked each day. Over 145,000 deaths could have been prevented in 2010 if adults without a high school diploma or GED had graduated from high school – roughly the number of preventable deaths among smokers who quit smoking.[482]

Adverse childhood events (ACEs) also put people at-risk for living shorter lives.[483] The seminal research study on ACEs was published in 1998 by a team led by Dr. Vincent Felitti at Kaiser Permanente. After studying 9,508 adult members of the health plan, the statistically significant conclusion was that exposure to childhood

WHITE NON-HISPANIC MIDLIFE MORTALITY FROM "DEATHS OF DESPAIR" IN THE U.S. BY EDUCATION

Ages 50-54, deaths by drugs, alcohol, and suicide

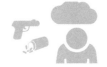

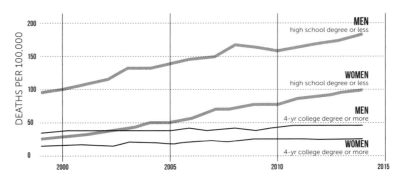

Source: Mortality and morbidity in the 21st century, Anne Case and Angus Deaton, Brookings Papers on Economic Activity, Spring 2017.

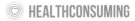 HEALTHCONSUMING

emotional, physical, or sexual abuse, and household dysfunction in childhood, were strong risk factors for early death. Subsequent research has re-confirmed this fact.[484]

In the U.S., people with lower incomes live shorter lives.[485] The Social Security Administration found that since the 1970s, Americans in the top-half of income distribution lived six years longer than people in the bottom half of income earners.

People in the U.S. earning lower incomes can afford less health insurance and health care services, and therefore less access to care. The Affordable Care Act began to reverse this trend through its inclusion of essential health benefits: before the ACA, patients with low-incomes were less likely to receive recommended preventive services such as cancer screening tests and immunizations. Before the implementation of the ACA, in 2012, one in five people age 50 to 75 with incomes of at least $75,000 had never been screened for colorectal cancer; 42 percent of the same-age people earning under $15,000 a year had never gotten screened for colorectal cancer, double the rate of wealthier older Americans.[486]

Education has also played a role in reversing the gains made in life expectancy in America for some middle-aged white men in America. These so-called deaths of despair have been associated among men in the U.S. with lower levels of educational attainment.[487]

Anne Case and Sir Angus Deaton of Princeton University coined the phrase "deaths of despair," observing a reversal in life expectancy among a cohort of middle-aged people. What's contributed most to this downturn are rising accidents, suicides, and drug overdoses.

There are two America's, Case and Deaton contend: one for people who have been to college, and another nation for people with a high school degree or less.

There is a cascading effect of social isolation, lessened job prospects and depressed wages for people with less education, based on Case and Deaton's analysis. This group of Americans has also seen a greater prevalence of declining family units, unstable marriages, eroding health status and, subsequently, rising death rates.

"It's about the collapse of the white middle class" in America, Case declared.[488]

This sad trend has led to the U.S. having the lowest life expectancy among the world's richest countries. The chart illustrates the continued improvement in life expectancy between 2000 and 2015 in France, Germany, the UK, Canada, Australia and Sweden. However, for the U.S., mortality rates for white non-Hispanic Americans age 45 to 54 rose at the same time as OECD nations' life spans improved.

MORTALITY RATE FOR 45-54 YEAR OLD WHITES IN THE U.S. ROSE WHILE FALLING IN OTHER WEALTHY COUNTRIES

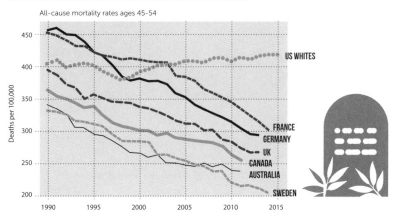

All-cause mortality rates ages 45-54

Source: Rising morbidity and mortality in midlife among white non-Hispanic Americans in the 21st century, Anne Case and Angus Deaton, Proceedings of the National Academy of Sciences, December 8, 2015

In this tragic context, remember that in 2018, the U.S. will have spent over 18 percent of the national economy on healthcare, in total and per person. Consider Germany, which allocates about 12 percent of the nation's GDP on healthcare. That is 6 percentage points lower than the U.S, proportion of GDP, equivalent to about $1 trillion in a year in the American economy. Note that U.S. national health spending is roughly the size of the entire German national economy – about $3.7 trillion $US in 2017.[489]

Case and Deaton believe this margin of greater U.S. healthcare spending has come from many places — especially from the wages of working-class Americans.

The hollowing out of the American middle class

In 1971, the majority of Americans were considered middle class in terms of income. By 2015, half of the U.S. population fell into the middle class, and the other half roughly split between upper and lower incomes. The Pew Research Center has tracked this phenomenon, in their report, *The American Middle Class Is Losing Ground.*

By 2015, income shifted from the middle class to upper income households, as the proportion of middle-income households declined from 62 percent of total families in America to only 43 percent. At the same time, median income for the shrinking middle-class fell by 4 percent from 2000 to 2014, and median household wealth in the group dropped more than one-fourth.[490]

Case and Deaton described this in their research on the roots of deaths of despair as the "upward redistribution" from lower income families to those in the upper income group, undermining the lives of American working families.

"Those without a bachelor's degree tumbled down the income tiers," the Pew researchers concluded. U.S. adults with no more than a high school diploma lost the most economic ground, which echoed Case and Deaton's calculations.

Expressed in terms of health and healthcare impacts, U.S., adults without a high school diploma are three times more likely to skip medical care compared with people who have a bachelor's degree or higher. Furthermore, adults with less than a high school education are twice as likely to lack a personal doctor.[491]

Wealth is health

The Social Security Administration found that since the 1970s, Americans in the top-half of income distribution live six years longer than people in the bottom half of incomes.[492]

After the ACA, there was a quantifiable improvement in health care access, as well as a ticking down of medical bad debt.[493]

Medical debt was the predominant factor in as many as one in four consumer bankruptcies in 2014.[494] But data analyzed by the American Bankruptcy Institute found a decline in bankruptcies following the rollout of the Affordable Care Act in 2011, illustrating the role that being health-insured can play as a social determinant of health and financial wellness.

"The first wealth is health," Ralph Waldo Emerson wrote in 1860 in his book, *The Conduct of Life*.[495] That quote is in a chapter called, "Power," in this context:

The first wealth is health. Sickness is poor-spirited, and cannot serve any one: it must husband its resources to live. But health or fullness answers its own ends, and has to spare, runs over, and inundates the neighborhoods and creeks of other men's necessities.

Most people appreciate that health is wealth. But for Americans, the inverse is also true: that wealth is a strong determinant of health.

The Great Recession of 2008 left a legacy of negative physical and financial health impacts. "While the relationship between homelessness and disease has long been common knowledge, the foreclosure crisis during the Great Recession taught us something new: the threat of foreclosure can contribute to illness before anyone loses their home," authors of a book warning about austerity's negative impact on health warned. Health risks from stress and struggles to deal with debt increased risks for depression by nine times,[496] and people skipped filling prescription drugs to make mortgage payments.[497]

Low ROI for health spending in the US

In 2020, national health expenditures in the U.S. are projected to exceed $4 trillion to cover 335 million Americans.[498]

AMERICANS SPEND TOO MUCH, SAVE TOO LITTLE, AND TAKE ON TOO MUCH DEBT

47% of Americans are spending more than or equal to their income

45% of Americans do not have enough savings to cover three months of living expenses

37% of Americans are not confident about their insurance coverage

36% of Americans are unable to pay all of their bills on time

30% of Americans say they have more debt than they can manage

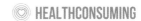

Source: Center for Financial Services Innovation, U.S. Financial Health Pulse: 2018 Baseline Survey Results, November 2018

HEALTHCONSUMING

Through the eyes of the American patient, now payor and health consumer, affordability ranks ahead of quality or access for health care.[499] Underneath affordability concerns is the fact that most consumers confess that they do not currently save for healthcare expenses. Furthermore, in 2018, consumer debt crept up toward Great Recession levels.

By 2018, most Americans agreed that the U.S. healthcare system was "in a state of crisis" in Gallup's survey.[500] That included 76 percent of Democrats and 71 percent of Republicans concurring that U.S. healthcare had major problems.

Americans' faith in the medical system eroded between 1975 and 2017. Each year, the Gallup Poll has asked U.S. adults about their faith in institutions: organized religion, the Supreme Court, Congress, organized labor, public schools, the military, and banks, along with the U.S. medical system. The question posed is, "how much confidence do you, yourself, have" in each institutional category − "a great deal, quite a lot, some or very little?"

In 1975, the first year Gallup asked the question, 80 percent of Americans had a lot of confidence in the nation's healthcare system. By 2017, that proportion fell by over half, to only 37 percent of people confident in American healthcare.[501]

Beyond financial and health insecurity, data insecurity

In the U.S., health security and financial wellness are inextricably linked. A third leg of the security stool is health data security, as discussed in the *Privacy* chapter.

In 1965, cybersecurity wasn't an issue when Lyndon Johnson signed amendments to the Social Security Act of 1935, Title XVIII and Title XIX, which provided for Medicare (hospital insurance for older Americans) and Medicaid (health care for lower-income Americans), respectively.

Since then, healthcare and other personal data that can be used for public health surveillance and precision medicine has gone digital. The promise of digital health tools – increasingly demanded by consumers and prescribed by physicians – is clear. Digital health is a cost driver/saver and can bring benefits to U.S. health care quality, access, and consumer engagement and empowerment.

But digital data are subject to leakages and attack. And today, cyber touches everything.

Most U.S. consumers are concerned about cyber incidents, but tend to underestimate the risk of breaches on their personal information. Just a handful of people were concerned about smart home-connected devices, along with personal laptops, smartphones, smart refrigerators and thermostats. Only 30 percent of U.S. consumers were concerned about having their medical records information breached, a 2018 Chubb survey found.[502]

In addition to medical record breaches, telehealth could also introduce risks to patients' privacy and data security.[503] HIPAA may need to be revisited in light of the growth of retail telehealth channels, which are generating consumer and patient data. As more telehealth visits are conducted in peoples' homes, their data could be used to infer consumer insights outside of the pure medical realm for which HIPAA protections were designed.

"We all benefit [from] the robust sharing of our data, because insights that may benefit all of us can be garnered. As we all know too well, there are also nefarious forces at play who aren't thinking how [to] use [data] for insights into human health, but how to use it for [manipulation]," Stanford faculty warned.[504]

Consumers will share their personal data if they are in charge of how it is used.[505] Consumers view their data as personal property, with most wanting the right to delete their online data.

The General Data Protection Regulation (GDPR), adopted in the European Union, set a new global gold standard for citizens' data protection. The over-arching goal of GDPR was to ensure the fundamental privacy rights of Europeans in the age of Big Data.[506]

The state of California took a page out of the GDPR, signing into law the Consumer Privacy Act of 2018 (CCPA). Beginning in 2020, the CCPA gives Californians several rights with respect to for-profit entities that conduct business in the state and collect residents' data: consumers' right to access personal data, the right to erase (delete) the data, the right to know what information has been collected, the right to know what information has been shared, and the right to opt out of personal data being sold – also known as, "the right to say 'no.'"[507]

"For data to remain the new oil," Deloitte suggested, "perhaps the benefits need to flow both ways."

Health data ownership as a civil right

Patients need and deserve the opportunity to control their health data, insisted a seminal essay published in October 2017 in *JAMA*, "The Pathway to Patient Data Ownership and Better Health."[508] While HIPAA affords people this right, it has been under-utilized by patients, and often made difficult by health care institutions.

In what was a two-page manifesto for patient data rights, attorney Katherine Mikk, technology analyst Harry Sleeper, and Dr. Eric Topol, a physician evangelist for digital health innovation, made the case that providing patients with their complete health data and control of it can help improve their health through increasing patient engagement and more informed, empowered self-care.

By 2019, though, the only state in America to grant health citizens legal ownership of their personal health information was New Hampshire. In the 49 other states, physician offices and hospitals controlled Americans' medical records. Even in New Hampshire, where state residents legally own their records, those patients don't necessarily have an easier path to obtaining those records. "The notion of 'ownership' there is likely more rhetorical than meaningful," Deven McGraw. Chief Regulatory Officer of Ciitizen, explained. [Note that McGraw was Deputy Director for Health Information Privacy at the Office of Civil Rights in the U.S. Department of Health and Human Services, responsible for enforcing HIPAA].

For the U.S. to be a high-performing health system, patients must trust that their information will be kept confidential.[509] That information is increasingly coming from outside traditional health data holders such as hospitals, physicians, health plans, and pharmacies – the usual HIPAA-covered entities. Today, consumers generate data via wearable technologies and health apps. A growing population is also conducting genetic testing via direct-to-consumer lab tests from Ancestry.com, 23andme, and other commercially-available gene-testing services.   Consumer-generated, genomic, and other data will mash up with patients' healthcare information for better diagnosis, treatment, and public health uses, increasingly applying artificial intelligence and machine learning technology.

But consumers' access to their records, and ability to control and monetize them, are elusive. "Patients lack access, but no one else seems to," two authors working in health and human rights wryly declared.[510] Third parties transacting business outside of HIPAA, especially data brokers and marketing agencies, are part of a multibillion-dollar industry that provides patient data. And patients, to date, have received little of the money generated by this huge and growing commercial enterprise.[511]

New models for patient health records are emerging with the explicit objective of giving consumers control of their personal health information, including the ability to share and monetize it. One such company is Ciitizen, with the bold mission of, "empowering the world's 7 billion citizens to have complete control of all of their health information, to share it easily with whomever, whenever and wherever they want," according to McGraw.

"Ciitizen takes advantage of the moral and legal right under HIPAA and other privacy laws for individuals to have copies of their health information; we gather all relevant information (not just what is available through portals) for patients and also normalize and standardize it, so that it can be populated into apps and other tools that will help people (or caregivers working on their behalf) get the best possible care," beginning with sicker patients, McGraw described. Ciitizen's goal is to enable patients to share information as they wish with health care providers, insurers, or researchers to support finding cures.

The company name, chosen by founder and CEO Anil Sethi, speaks to the last three line-items on a chart that Dr. Topol included in his book, *The Patient Will See You Now*, explaining the criticality of patients controlling their data:[512]

1   You can handle the truth
2   You need to own your data; it should be a civil right
3   It could save your life.

"As patients, we must secure access to our health data, have the opportunity to learn from it, and the freedom to share it with whomever we wish. As Americans, we deserve this," Hugo Campos wrote upon the occasion of receiving an award for being a White House Champion of Change for Precision Medicine.[613]

One benefit of patient control of their health data is the ability to monetize it — that is, sell, it. Start-up companies are working out business models to enable patients to sell their genetic and health data.[514] As discussed in the *Digital Health* chapter, patients are growing to realize the value of their data in research, both for basic science and in for-profit life science companies. Bio-brokers are organizing to sell or "rent" consumers' data to research institutes, universities and drug companies, with revenue going to patients.

Nebula Genomics developed a business for consumers to

purchase a DNA testing kit, submit their sample, receive information back about ancestry and disease risks, secure the personal data via blockchain technology, and earn compensation for sharing their information. The data security and compensation features distinguish Nebula Genomics from other direct-to-consumer genetic test kits such as Ancestry.com and 23andme.

During the holiday gifting season of 2017, Ancestry.com sold about 1.5 million testing kits.

"That's like 2,000 gallons of saliva—enough to fill a modest above-ground swimming pool with the genetic history of every person in the city of Philadelphia," according to *WIRED* magazine's observation that, "Ancestry's genetic testing kits are heading for your stocking this year."[515]

A self-described "Match.com for patient insights," Savvy, organized as a public-benefit corporation, is a cooperative owned collectively by patients that contribute their data to the coop. Savvy was founded by two patients (one diagnosed with juvenile diabetes, and one managing cystic fibrosis) who wanted to share their data and patient experience with researchers and pharma, as a platform to enable patients to get paid for their data. "Connecting patients with the medical industry is a lucrative market," co-founder Jen Horonjeff realized. "We didn't want to make something that would just be a small group of people benefiting off a bunch of patients doing the work, because that's the way the power dynamic in healthcare has always been," she recognized.

Shifting the healthcare power dynamic: Americans' right to health citizenship

In a democracy, the decision to extend universal health care is a choice for the body politic – in the U.S., American voters and taxpayers who have morphed into payors.

The facts are that Americans pay more and get less for health care; individual and population health outcomes depend heavily on one's ZIP code and geography; health disparities between the wealthy and not-so-rich are exacerbating; the one-in-five dollars allocated to sick-care in the U.S. crowds out other investments in America's human capital and infrastructure; and, while digital technologies hold great promise to improve quality, precision, and access for healthcare, the volume, velocity, and variety of data these tools generate are a rich target for hackers and data brokers that can exclude patients from benefiting from the value of their data.

In the U.S., we need to imagine and build a uniquely American universal healthcare system, a solution that increases quality, decreases costs, conserves the resilience of our health care workers, and bolsters favorable individual and public health outcomes.

Public health is personal health at the ZIP code level. See the map of life expectancy in Philadelphia, illustrating that if you reside northeast of Temple University, you are likely to live 20 fewer years than residents who live in Olde City near the Liberty Bell and Independence Hall.

Independence Hall is where the Founding Fathers convened to get to a consensus about life, liberty, pursuits of happiness, and men and women being created equal. Do Americans today believe these concepts extend to health?

The evidence in terms of what we spend *vis-à-vis* outcomes and the burden of disease demonstrate that "no," we do not.

SHORT DISTANCES TO LARGE GAPS IN HEALTH

This life expectancy map of Philadelphia shows a 20-year difference in life expectancy only a few miles apart.

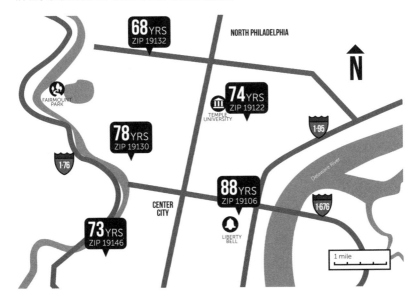

Source: Robert Wood Johnson Foundation, VCU, Center on Society and Health

The longer we avoid facing the gaps of health disparities, over-spending, and out-moded healthcare delivery models, the more at-risk we put the body politic – both the "body" physical and the "political" chasm between Americans. The result in delaying greater attention to the social determinants of health and digital tools to scale services from where and to whom they are needed will be greater mortality from deaths of despair, and quality of life for causes that are amenable to change through social investments and peoples' lifestyle changes.

We return to Independence Hall and the Founding Fathers as they met in secrecy to deliberate the Constitutional Convention of 1787. After the proceedings concluded, Mrs. Powell of Philadelphia asked Benjamin Franklin, "Well, Doctor, what have we got, a Republic or a Monarchy?"

Ben Franklin responded, "You have a Republic...if you can keep it."[516]

Addressing healthcare reform at the fundamental level of universal access will help America keep her Republic, politically, socially, and fiscally fit.

Most Americans know the Declaration's unalienable rights of life, liberty, and the pursuit of happiness. The conclusion of that paragraph in the document speaks to, "organizing [its] powers in such form, as to them shall seem most likely to affect their Safety and Happiness."

"The phrase 'safety and happiness' was an 18th-century update of the ancient Roman idea that the supreme guide for all political decision-making was "*salus populi*," the health and well-being of the people."[517]

"If we are connected to everyone else by six degrees and we can influence them up to three degrees, then one way to think about ourselves is that each of us can reach about halfway to everyone else on the planet," Christakis and Fowler wrote.

What a uniquely United States of Health could look like

As health citizens, people living in America would be covered by a uniquely United States for Health:

- Universal access to quality healthcare and preventive services for all

- Care accessible in settings convenient to and safe for patients and consumers, leveraging modern digital technologies that optimize physicians' and nurses' workflow and patient/user-centered design principles

- Data under the control of patients, and a privacy policy upgrade

- Greater allocation of resources on evidence-based prevention and social determinants of health, away from downstream sick-care

Public policy-making that bakes "health" into policies across the cabinet levels beyond the Department of Health and Human Services, with examples shown in the table.

Opportunities to "Bake Health" Into U.S. Public Policy

Cabinet Department	Examples of "baked-in" health policies
Agriculture	Nutrition programs, food security
Education	Early childhood education, training for the knowledge economy
Energy	Utility access for low-income consumers
Housing	Enforced regulation of safe buildings
Interior	Clean air, clean water regulations and enforcement
Justice	Criminal justice reform
Labor	Job retraining, job security, fair wages in the gig economy
Transportation	More active transportation incentives; public and private transportation to support health citizens' engagement

Furthermore, independent agencies have roles to play in addressing social determinants of health:

- The Consumer Financial Protection Bureau, for medical debt and medical bill collections
- The Environmental Protection Agency, for clean air and clean water

◉ The Federal Communications Commission, for broadband access and net neutrality, and

◉ The Federal Trade Commission, for antitrust and privacy regulation.

As health citizens, Americans would have rights and responsibilities. Some of these could be:

◉ The right to high quality healthcare delivery
◉ The right to elect representatives in government to promote policies and laws that support health outcomes
◉ The right to clean air, clean water, safe food, and broadband connectivity
◉ The right to own and control our data
◉ The responsibility to take care of ourselves, as part of our local and national community of fellow/sister health citizens
◉ The responsibility to be informed on health care issues
◉ The responsibility to participate in our democracy.

Americans brought modern democracy to the world, cured polio, and put a man on the moon, all through mindful and strategic investments in human capital and collective well-being.

Why have we chosen to pay so much to get so little in return in the form of worse outcomes, health inequities, and lack of coverage for all Americans?

Americans can choose to build a better healthcare system for the nation.

Home is not just where the heart is: it's our health hub

If fully realized, this new deal in health care should evolve into people owning, not "renting," their health, as Esther Dyson has said. The concept of self-health goes back at least to a 1919 guide titled *Self-Health as a Habit*, written by a British athlete named

Eustace Miles. She wrote in the book's forward,

To-day, more than ever, there is demanded, from every member of the Empire, greater all-round efficiency and economy....Health is a duty, and should be added to our list of our duties towards God and our duties towards our Neighbour.

Interestingly, a century before Christakis and Fowler's research into the impact of social networks on our health, Miles talked about true health being, "infectious."[518] In Miles' early 20th century world, self-care was understood to be a civic responsibility.[519] And, Miles insisted, that self-health was the highest form of health: not dependent on drugs, inoculations, and hygiene.

Ultimately, our homes and bodies can evolve into our personal health hubs, informed by our data (secured, perhaps by blockchain, and under our control). We will be guided, educated and supported, through opt-in and request, by concierges (digital and human, alike) who could be doctors, nurses, health coaches, pharmacists, community health workers, genetic counselors, peers and other roles we may not be able to conceive of in this moment.

So many of the technologies to build our home health hubs are commercially available or in development. Technology won't be the barrier to bringing our health home. Public policy, lagging regulations, political will and personal commitment are the obstacles to people engaging in a new deal for self-care. American patients – consumers, caregivers, all – have the collective influence and choice to make this vision real.

Endnotes

REFERENCES

[1] U.S. General Services Administration, Federal Register Division, National Archives and Records Service. Public Papers of the Presidents of the United States, Book 1, Ronald Reagan, 1984. Message to the Congress Transmitting Proposed Health Care Incentives Reform Legislation, February 28, 1983

[2] The Associated Press-NORC Center for Public Affairs Research. New Year, Same Priorities: The Public's Agenda for 2018, Issue Brief, November 30, 2017

[3] Pollack R, Tavenner M. When your medication costs more than your mortgage. The Hill, December 31, 2017

[4] Fox M. Rising health-care costs a "huge threat" to US economy: Cleveland Clinic's Toby Cosgrove. CNBC, January 30, 2018

[5] Stempel J. Buffett: Health care "tapeworm" drags on economy. Reuters, March 1, 2010

[6] Olson J. Mayo to give preference to privately insured patients over Medicaid patients, March 15, 2017

[7] Luckstein K. Statement from Mayo Clinic on patient appointment concerns. Mayo Clinic press release, March 17, 2017

[8] Cuckler GA, Sisko AM, Poisal JA, Keehan SP, Smith SD, Madison AJ, Wolfe CJ, Hardesty JC. National Health Expenditure Projections, 2017-26: Despite Uncertainty, Fundamentals Primarily Drive Spending Growth. Health Affairs, March 2018

[9] Centers for Disease Control, National Center for Health Statistics. Mortality in the United States, 2015. NCHS Data Brief, No. 267, December 2016

[10] OECD. Health at a Glance 2018. How does the United States compare? June 2018

[11] OECD. Heatlh at a Glance, 2018

[12] Deaton A, Case A. An Update on Rising Mortality Rates Among White, Working-Class Americans. Wall Street Journal, November 19, 2017

[13] Preston S, Vierboom YC, Stokes A. The role of obesity in exceptionally slow US mortality improvement. PNAS, January 30, 2018

[14] Kaiser Family Foundation. Kaiser Health Tracking Poll: October 2015. October 28, 2015

[15] Brookings Institution analysis of Consumer Expenditure Survey, Labor Department

[16] Nadar AB. "Godmother" Revisited. Health Affairs. May 2008 vol. 27, no. 3, 901

[17] Edelman. Health Engagement Barometer: Health Influence in the Era of Public Engagement, 2008

[18] Strategy&/PwC. The birth of the health care consumer, October 14, 2014

[19] comScore, comScore Reports March 2015 U.S. Smartphone Subscriber Market Share, May 7, 2015

[20] Pew Research Center, American Trends Panel Survey, October 3-27 2014

[21] U.S. Government Accountability office, Broadband: Intended Outcomes and Effectiveness of Efforts to Address Adoption Barriers Are Unclear, June 2015

[22] Parks Associates, Smart Home Platforms for Health, July 2015

[23] Packaged Facts. Health-Conscious and Ingredient-Aware Consumers Want Food Nutritional Labeling to Be "Clean" as Well as Seen, May 21, 2015

[24] Prevention, Rodale and FMI. Shopping for Health, 2014

[25] Strom S. Employing Dietitians Pays Off for Supermarkets, New York Times, August 24, 2012

[26] FMI, 2014 Report on Retailer Contributions to Health and Wellness

[27] IRI survey of U.S. households, 2015

[28] Centers for Disease Control and Prevention, National Center for Health Statistics, Characteristics of Office-based Physician Visits, 2016

[29] Carger E, Westen D. Robert Wood Johnson Foundation. A New Way to Talk about the Social Determinants of Health, January 1, 2010

[30] Moody's. US Healthcare Reform: Three Risks Reduce Credit Positives for Not-for-Profit Hospitals, March 27, 2014. Quote attributed to Daniel Steingart of Moody's

[31] WEGO Health and Sarasohn-Kahn J. The Empowered Patient and the Endangered Wallet. Survey, February 2018

[32] Cramer Maria, Cote J. A horrific injury. A heroic rescue effort. And a desperate plea: Please don't call the ambulance, it costs too much. Boston Globe, July 2, 2018

[33] Jones JM. U.S. Concerns About Healthcare High; Energy, Unemployment Low. Gallup, March 26, 2018

[34] Employee Benefits Research Institute. Workers Rank Health Care as the Most Critical Issue in the United States. EBRI Notes, Vol. 39, No. 1, January 2018

[35] WestHealth Institute and NORC. New Survey Finds Large Number of People Skipping Necessary Medical Care Because of Cost. More Americans fear medical bills than they do serious illness. Press release, March 26, 2018

[36] American Psychological Association. Uncertainty About Healthcare: Stress in America poll, January 24, 2018

[37] TransUnion Healthcare. TransUnion Healthcare survey finds consumers are concerned about rising health insurance rates for 2017. June 2015

[38] Health Care Incentives Improvement Institute (HCI3) and Catalyst for Payment Report (CPR). 2016 Report Card on State Transparency Laws, July 2016

[39] Newman D, Parente S, Barrette E, Kennedy K. Prices for Common Medical Services Vary Substantially Among the Commercially Insured. Health Affairs, May 2016

[40] Centers for Disease Control and Prevention, National Center for Health Statistics. National Vital Statistics Reports – Births: Preliminary Data for 2015, Volume 65, Number 3, June 2, 2016

[41] Xu X, Gariepy A, Lundsberg LS, Sheth SS, Pettker CM, Krumholz HM, Illuzzi JL. Wide Variation Found in Hospital Facility Costs For Maternity Stays Involving Low-Risk Childbirth. Health Affairs, July 2015

[42] Aiello M. Maternity Campaign Focuses on Luxury, Not Babies. HealthLeaders, May 11, 2016

[43] Alegeus. 2016 Alegeus Healthcare 'Moments of Truth' Research Report, July 2016

[44] Rosenberg T. Shopping for Health Care: A Fledgling Craft. New York Times, April 12, 2016

[45] Chernew M, Cooper Z, Larsen-Hallock E, Morton FS. Are Health Care Services Shoppable? Evidence from the Consumption of Lower-Limb MRI Scans. National Bureau of Economic Research, July 2018

[46] Prager E. Will People Price Shop for Healthcare? KelloggInsight, January 4, 2018. Based on Consumer Responsiveness to Simple Health Care Prices: Evidence From Tiered Hospital Networks, September 21, 2017

[47] Alegeus. 2016 Healthcare Consumerism Index, June 21, 2016

[48] Mangan D. How bad are we at buying health insurance? Very, very bad. CNBC, May 15, 2015

[49] Hanauer DA, Zheng K, Singer DC, Gebremariam A, Davis MM. Public awareness, perception, and use of online physician rating sites. JAMA, 2014:311(7):734-735

[50] Lagu T, Metayer K, Moran M, Ortiz L, Priya A, Goff S, Lindenauer PK. Website Characteristics and Physician Reviews on Commercial Physician-Rating Websites - JAMA, February 21, 2017, 317(7): 766-768

[51] Edelman. The Edelman Health Engagement Barometer, 2009

[52] Turunen E, Hiilamo H. Health effects of indebtedness: a systematic review. BMC Public Health, 22 May 2014

[53] Gutman A, Garon T, Hogarth J, Schneider R. Understanding and Improving Consumer Financial Health in America," Center for Financial Services Innovation (CFSI), March 24, 2015

[54] Moody's. Three risks reduce credit positives of Affordable Care Act for not-for-profit hospitals, 27 March 2014

[55] Consumer Finance Protection Bureau. Consumer credit reports: A study of medical and non-medical collections. December 11, 2014

[56] Hamel L., et al. The Burden of Medical Debt: Results from the Kaiser Family Foundation/New York Times Medical Bills Survey, January 2016

[57] U.S. Bureau of Economic Analysis, Personal Saving Rate [PSAVERT], retrieved from FRED, Federal Reserve Bank of St. Louis; https://fred.stlouisfed.org/series/PSAVERT, December 5, 2018

[58] Goldstein S. Nearly half don't have the cash to pay for a $400 emergency, Fed survey finds. MarketWatch, May 19, 2017

[59] Kaiser Family Foundation. 2018 Employer Health Benefits Survey, October 3, 2018

[60] Cuckler GA, Sisko AM, Poisal JA, Keehan SP, Smith SD, Madison AJ, Wolfe CJ, Hardesty JC. National Health Expenditure Projections, 2017-26: Despite Uncertainty, Fundamentals Primarily Drive Spending Growth. Health Affairs, March 2018

[61] PBS News Hour. Maker of $1,000 hepatitis C pill was focused on profits, not patients, report finds. December 1, 2015

[62] Andrews M. Medical Debt Is Top Reason Consumers Hear from Collection Agencies. Kaiser Health News and NPR, January 24, 2017

[63] Consumer Financial Protection Bureau. Consumer credit reports: A study of medical and non-medical collections. December 2014

[64] Board of Governors of the Federal Reserve System, Report on the Economic Well-Being of U.S. Households in 2016, May 2017

[65] Blau M. In the state with the highest medical debt, it's the middle class who carries the burden. STAT, March 24, 2017

[66] Karpman M, Long SK. 9.4 Million Fewer Families Are Having Problems Paying

Medical Bills. Urban Institute Health Policy Center, May 21, 2015
[67] Jackson C. One in Five Americans Could Not Afford to Pay an Unexpected Medical Bill Without Accumulating Some Debt. Ipsos Public Affairs, March 21, 2017
[68] Seifert RW, Rukavina M. Bankruptcy Is The Tip Of A Medical-Debt Iceberg, Health Affairs, March 2006
[69] Samuel L. Inside the medical debt charity that John Oliver just made famous. STAT, June 6, 2016
[70] Gould E. The State of American Wages 2016. Economic Policy Institute, March 9, 2017
[71] Gould E. The State of American Wages 2017. Economic Policy Institute, March 1, 2018
[72] Black Book Research. Providers Driven to Implement Patient Centric Financial Solutions as Consumer Payment Responsibility Skyrockets 29 Percent, October 24, 2017
[73] Lagasse J. Healthcare providers explore no-interest loans to help patients pay for care, say move cuts bad debt. Healthcare Finance News, July 6, 2016
[74] HealthFirst Financial. HealthFirst Financial Patient Survey, September 12, 2017
[75] Luthra S. Hospital bank loans leave patients vulnerable. Kaiser Health News, February 21, 2018
[76] Kaiser Family Foundation. The Burden of Medical Debt: Results of the Kaiser Family Foundation/New York Times Medical Bills Survey, January 5, 2016
[77] Barclay E. The Sick Turn To Crowd Funding To Pay Medical Bills, October 24, 2012
[78] Jopson B. Why are so many Americans crowdfunding their healthcare? Financial Times, January 11, 2018
[79] Quartz Index, June 15, 2017
[80] Pew Research Center. Shared, Collaborative and On-Demand: The New Digital Economy, May 19, 2016
[81] Jopson
[82] Reindl JC. Hospital denies woman's heart transplant, recommends 'fundraising' to pay for it. Detroit Free Press, November 26, 2018
[83] Adams S. Free Market Philanthropy: GoFundMe Is Changing The Way People Give To Causes Big And Small. Forbes, October 19, 2016
[84] Experian. Patient-Engagement Bundle. Accessed March 26, 2017 at: https://www.experian.com/assets/healthcare/brochures/patient-engagement-bundle.pdf
[85] Young MJ, Scheinberg E. The Rise of Crowdfunding for Medical Care Promises and Perils. JAMA, March 23, 2017
[86] Hopkins BR, Kirkpatrick A. The Law of Fundraising. 5th ed. New York, NY: Wiley Online Library; 2013
[87] Kaiser Family Foundation and Health Research & Education Trust. Employer Health Benefits: 2017 Summary of Findings, September 19, 2017
[88] Altman D. The Next Big Debate in Health Care. Wall Street Journal, June 30, 2016. From Kaiser Family Foundation analysis of Truven Health Analytics MarketScan Commercial Claims and Encounters Database, 2004-2014; Bureau of Labor Statistics, Seasonally Adjusted Data form the Current Employment Statistics Survey, 2004-2014
[89] Sussman AL. 5 Things to Know About Health-Care Spending in the U.S. Wall Street Journal, August 25, 2016
[90] Sussman AL. Burden of Healthcare Costs Moves to the Middle Class. Wall Street Journal, August 25, 2016
[91] Kaiser Family Foundation. The Burden of Medical Debt – Results from the Kaiser Family Foundation/New York Times Medical Bills Survey, January 2016
[92] Alegeus. 2016 Alegeus Healthcare Consumerism Index, June 22, 2016
[93] Girod CS, Hart SK, Weitz S. Milliman Medical Index 2018, May 2018

[94] Kaiser Family Foundation. The Burden of Medical Debt – Results from the Kaiser Family Foundation/New York Times Medical Bills Survey, January 2016

[95] Griffen P. Waiting to Feel Better: Survey Reveals Cost Delays Timely Care. Earnin website, October 23, 2018

[96] Tepper T. Most Americans don't have enough savings to cover a $1K emergency. Bankrate website, January 18, 2018

[97] Dhaliwal KK, King-Shier K, Manns BJ, Hemmelgarn BR, Stone JA, Campbell DJT. Exploring the impact of financial barriers on secondary prevention of heart disease. BMC Cardiovascular Disorders, 2017 17:61

[98] Campbell DJT, Manns BJ, Weaver RG, Hemmelgarn BR, King-Shier KM, Sanmartin C. Financial barriers and adverse clinical outcomes among patients with cardiovascular-related chronic diseases: a cohort study. BMC Medicine, December 2017, 15:33

[99] Gallup. U.S. Women More Likely Than Men to Put Off Medical Tratment, December 6, 2017

[100] Prescription Justice. 45 Million Americans Forego Medications Due to Costs, New Analysis Shows – 9 Times the Rate of the UK, February 6, 2017

[101] Skinner G. As Drug Prices Increase, Quality of Life Goes Down. Consumer Reports, June 21, 2016

[102] CBS News. The Cost of Cancer Drugs, October 5, 2014. Accessed at http://www.cbsnews.com/news/cost-of-cancer-drugs-60-minutes-lesley-stahl-health-care/ on February 13, 2017

[103] Shankaran V, Jolly S, et al. Risk Factors for Financial Hardship in Patients Receiving Adjuvant Chemotherapy for Colon Cancer: A Population-Based Exploratory Analysis. Journal of Clinical Oncology. 30; 14(May 2012), 1608-1614

[104] Ramsey S, Blough D, et al. Washington State Cancer Patients Found to Be At Greater Risk for Bankruptcy Than People Without A Cancer Diagnosis. Health Affairs, May 15, 2013

[105] Ramsey SD, Bansal A, et al. Financial Insolvency as a Risk Factor for Early Mortality Among Patients With Cancer. Journal of Clinical Oncology, 2016 March 20; 34(9): 980-986

[106] Stahl L. The Cost of Cancer Drugs. CBS News, 60 Minutes, October 5, 2014

[107] Dobkin C, Finkelstein A, Kluender R, Notowidigdo MJ. Myth and Measurement – The Case of Medical Bankruptcies. New England Journal of Medicine, 378;12, March 22, 2018

[108] Gilligan AM, Alberts DS, Roe DJ, Skrepnek GH. Death or Debt? National Estimates of Financial Toxicity in Persons with Newly-Diagnosed Cancer. The American Journal of Medicine, June 12, 2018

[109] People magazine. Passages, September 12, 2016

[110] MAD magazine. Reasons Why the Price of EpiPens Increased, August 24, 2016

[111] Kodjak A and Martin M. Mother Calls EpiPen Price Hike 'A Matter of Life and Death." August 27, 2016

[112] CNBC. Full interview with Mylan CEO Heather Bresch on drug pricing, Trump. March 3, 2017

[113] Murphy T. CVS cuts the price of a generic EpiPen competitor in half. January 12, 2017

[114] Rice C. Prescriptions jump for EpiPen alternatives, athenaInsight, March 3, 2017

[115] Sanger-Katz M. Even Insured Can Face Crushing Medical Debt, Study Finds, New York Times, January 5, 2016

[116] Aflac. 2016 Aflac Open Enrollment Survey, October 4, 2016

[117] Brand Keys. 2018 Loyalty Leaders, September 12, 2018

[118] Temkin Group. 2018 Temkin Experience Ratings, March 2018

[119] Merritt Hawkins. Survey: Physician Appointment Wait Times Up 30% From 2014, March 20, 2017

[120] TIME. December 25, 2006

[121] Pew Research Center. A third of Americans live in a household with three or more smartphones. May 25, 2017

[122] EY. Consumers on Board – How to copilot the multichannel journey, July 2014

[123] Accenture. Virtual Health: The Untapped Opportunity to Get the Most out of Healthcare, February 9, 2017

[124] Werle M, McGuire R. Nearly One-Half of U.S. Households Now Prime Members. Kantar Retail IQ, 17 January 2018

[125] Bezos J. 2017 Letter to Shareholders, April 18 2018

[126] Franck T. Amazon Prime subscribers will more than double to 275 million in the next decade, Citi says. CNBC, September 10, 2018

[127] Consumer Intelligence Research Partners, LLC. Amazon Prime Reaches 85 Million U.S. Members, July 6, 2017

[128] Laughlin S. The In-Store Retail Imperative: A Return to Relationships. THINK Blog, IBM, January 27, 2017

[129] Aflac. Aflac 2016 Workforces Report and Survey, October 2016

[130] Griswold A. Even Amazon is surprised by how much people love Alexa. Quartz, February 4, 2018

[131] Invoca. The Rise of Voice. White paper, November 16, 2017

[132] Coombs B. Alexa's best skill could be home health-care assistant. CNBC, August 9, 2017

[133] BabyCenter. 71 Percent of Today's Parents Own at Least One 'Internet of Things' Device & Three-Quarters of Those Without IoT are Interested and Want to Learn More, According to BabyCenter Research. Press release, January 4, 2017

[134] Comstock J. GoodRx launches Alexa app for finding the cheapest prescription drugs. MobiHealthNews, December 14, 2017

[135] Siwicki B. AI voice assistants have officially arrived in healthcare. Healthcare IT News, February 01, 2018

[136] Anders G. Amazon Purchases 40% Stake in Web Upstart Drugstore.com. Wall Street Journal, February 25, 1999

[137] Ross C. Amazon failed to disrupt the prescription drug business with Drugstore.com. Could a second try succeed? STAT, April 26, 2018

[138] Ouchi MS. Amazon, drugstore.com to dissolve partnership. Seattle Times, February 1, 2012

[139] Cook J. Amazon patents new Alexa feature that knows when you're ill and offers you medicine, The Telegraph, 9 October 2018

[140] PYMNTS. Amazon Rolls Out Private-Label Vitamins, March 6, 2017

[141] Smart B. Barbershop health clinic provides free medical care in Wilmington. WECT, December 18, 2017

[142] Balls-Berry J, Dacy LC, Bals J. "Heard It through the Grapevine:" The Black Barbershop as a Source of Health Information. Hektoen International – A Journal of Medical Humanities, Volume 7, Issue 3, Summer 2015

[143] Frost K. M&S Launches Drop-In Sessions to Support Those Suffering from Stress and Anxiety. Country Living, March 14, 2017

[144] Levin, J. Partnerships between the faith-based and medical sectors: Implications for preventive medicine and public health. Preventive medicine reports Vol. 4 344-50. 27 Jul. 2016

[145] Idler EI. Religion as a Social Determinant of Public Health. Oxford Scholarship Online, September 2014

[146] The National Academies of Sciences, Engineering and Medicine. Faith – Health Collaboration to Improve Population Health: A Workshop Roundtable on Population Health Improvement. Shaw University, Raleigh, NC, March 22, 2018

[147] Szeltner M, Van Horn C, Zukin C. Diminished Lives and Futures: A Portrait of America in the Great-Recession Era, Rutgers University, John J. Heldrich Center for Workforce Development. Worktrends report, February 2013

[148] Communispace and Ogilvy & Mather. Eyes Wide Open, Wallet Half Shut: the Emerging Post-Recession Consumer Consciousness, March 2010

[149] Althouse BM, Allem J-P, Childers MA, Dredze M, Ayers JW. Population Health Concerns During the United States' Great Recession, American Journal of Preventive Medicine, Volume 46 , Issue 2 , 166 - 170

[150] Ogilvy. Eyes Wide Open, Wallet Half Shut: The Emerging Post-Recession Consumer Consciousness, March 15, 2010

[151] Forrester. Do Your Customers Want to Telephone You For Service? April 6, 2010

[152] Nuance Communications. Survey Shows: Majority of Consumers Frustrated with Web Self-Service, Want a "Human" Touch, December 16, 2013

[153] Trevail C, Austin M, Schlack JW, Lerman K. The Brands That Make Customers Feel Respected. Harvard Business Review, November 1, 2016

[154] Centers for Disease Control and Prevention. National Ambulatory Medical Care Survey: 2012 Summary Tables, January 11, 2016

[155] Riley RW. Health Starts Where We Learn. Robert Wood Johnson Foundation, 19 October 2010

[156] Edelman. Edelman Health Engagement Barometer 2010, April 2010

[157] Strategy& (PwC). The birth of the healthcare consumer, October 28, 2014

[158] Oliver Wyman. The New Front Door to Healthcare is Here, March 17, 2016

[159] Poon SJ, Schuur JD, Mehrotra A. Trends in Visits to Acute Care Venues for Treatment of Low-Acuity Conditions in the United States From 2008-2015. JAMA Internal Medicine, October 2018

[160] Weinick RM, Burns RM, Mehrotra A. Many Emergency Department Visits Could Be Managed At Urgent Care Centers And Retail Clinics. Health Affairs, September 2010 vol 29 no 9 1630-1636

[161] Charland T. The Window May Be Closing: 2019 Mid-Year Review. Merchant Medicine, July 16, 2018

[162] Mehrotra A. The Evolving Role of Retail Clinics. RAND, November 10, 2016

[163] Shrank WH, Krumme AA, Tong AY, Spettell CM, Matlin OS, Sussman A, Brennan TA, Chourdhry NK. Quality of Care at Retail Clinics for 3 Common Conditions. The American Journal of Managed Care, October 2014, Vol. 20, No. 10

[164] Carroll AE. The Undeniable Convenience and Reliability of Retail Health Clinics. New York Times, April 12, 2016

[165] Calandra R. Chronic Illness New Battleground for Retail Clinics, Primary Care Physicians. Managed Care, June 2016

[166] Merchant Medicine. 2017 Urgent Care Benchmark Report

[167] Urgent Care Association of America. Certified Urgent Care (CUC) Program criteria, 2016-2017

[168] Snowbeck C. UnitedHealth's Optum unit makes big push into urgent care in Minnesota. Minneapolis Star-Tribune, September 13, 2016

[169] Landro L. Traditional Providers Get Into the Urgent-Care Game. Wall Street Journal, March 20, 2016

[170] Wilson L. Data Exchange Rises in Importance for Urgent Care Providers. Health Data Management, August 25, 2016

[171] One Medical press release. One Medical Announces up to $350M Investment to Expand National Footprint. August 22, 2018

[172] Drug Store News. RxImpact: Pharmacy, the face of neighborhood health care in America. March 2017

[173] Drug Store News. Profile of leading pharmacy retailers, April 27, 2015

[174] Fein A. The 2017 Economic Report on U.S. Pharmacies and Pharmacy Benefit Managers. Pembroke Consulting, Drug Channels Institute, January 2017

[175] Fortune. Fortune 500. June 6, 2016

[176] Brenan M. Nurses Keep Healthy Lead as Most Honest, Ethical Profession. Gallup, December 26, 2017

[177] Anderson SC. See the face of neighborhood health care. Drug Store News, March 2017

[178] The Network for Excellence in Health Innovation. Thinking Outside the Pillbox: A System-wide Approach to Improving Patient Medication Adherence for Chronic Disease. August 12, 2009

[179] PrescribeWellness. PrescribeWellness 2017 Vaccination and Preventive Care Survey: 89 Percent of Americans Feel Shingles Vaccination Is a Priority. Business Wire, March 23, 2017

[180] National Governors Association. The Expanding Role of Pharmacists in a Transformed Health Care System. NGA Paper, January 13, 2015

[181] Brohan M. Digital drugstores are the new shopping malls of healthcare. Digital Commerce 360, February 14, 2018

[182] Business Wire. Amazon to Acquire PillPack, June 28, 2018

[183] J.D. Power. U.S. Pharmacies Raise Bar for Customer Satisfaction, Setting Stage for Fierce Competition in Digital/Mail Order Market, J.D. Power Finds. Press release, August 28, 2018

[184] MMGY. Portrait of American Travelers 2018-2019, June 2018

[185] Eckhardt GM, Husemann KC. The Growing Business of Helping Customers Slow Down. Harvard Business Review, December 7, 2018

[186] Raphael R. Burned-Out Americans Are Helping Wellness Tourism Flourish. Fast Company, October 29, 2016

[187] Gibson A. Three Days At Cal-a-Vie. Forbes, December 21, 2017

[188] SpaFinder Wellness 365 survey

[189] Kanowitz S. Hotels put bigger focus on fitness with in-room equipment. The Washington Post, May 31, 2017

[190] Petersen A. Luxury Hotels Latest Amenities Are Brand-Name Fitness Classes. Wall Street Journal, June 24, 2015

[191] Fox JT/ Hotels see value in wellness investment. Global Wellness Institute, February 14, 2018

[192] Shallcross J. At Even Hotels, the Guest Rooms Double as Gyms. Conde Nast Traveler, August 13, 2015

[193] Christoff J. Hyatt Making Major Investment in Miraval Expansion. TravelPulse, February 19, 2018

[194] Powell L. Hyatt's New Wellness Exec Talks Strategy. Skift, December 18, 2018

[195] Zemler E. Hotels join forces with popular fitness brands. USA Today, October 3, 2016

[196] Kalosh A. New Regent wellness program pairs excursions with Canyon Ranch treatments. Seatrade Cruise News, March 27, 2017

[197] Seabourn press release. Seabourn Announces Content Rich "Wellness Cruises with Dr. Andrew Weil" Bound for Alaska and Greece in 2018, November 20, 2017

[198] Levine IS. Blue World Voyages: A New Cruise Line For Health And Wellness Enthusiasts. Forbes, July 11, 2018

[199] International Health, Racquet and Sportsclub Association. 2018 IHRSA Health Club Consumer Report, March 2018

[200] ZOOM Media. 2018 Generation Active Survey, August 16, 2018

[201] Rubin R. House Panel Passes Tax Break for Gym Memberships, Exercise Classes. Wall Street Journal, July 12, 2018

[202] Market Force Information. US Health & Beauty: Consumer Experiences & Competitive Benchmarks, January 2017

[203] Schroeder EC, Welk GJ, Franke WD, Lee D-c. Associations of Health Club Membership with Physical Activity and Cardiovascular Health. PLOS, January 20, 2017

[204] American Heart Association. YMCA and American Heart Association Join Forces to Improve Blood Pressure Control, press release, March 29, 2018

[205] Alva ML, Hoerger TJ, Jeyaraman R, Amico P, Rojas-Smith L. Impact of the YMCA Of The USA Diabetes Prevention Program On Medicare Spending and Utilization. Health Affairs, Vol. 36, No. 3, March 2017

[206] YMCA of Greater Louisville. YMCA of Greater Louisville and Charter Partners

Announce Comprehensive Health Facility. Press release, September 25, 2017
[207] Chinn V. Philip Morris property being developed. WDRB, October 27, 2010
[208] Quinnipiac University. U.S. Voters Believe Comey More Than Trump. Quinnipiac University National Poll Finds; Support For Marijuana Hits New High, April 26, 2018
[209] National Conference of State Legislatures. State Medical Marijuana Laws, November 8, 2018
[210] Global Market Insights. U.S. Medical Marijuana Market, Aug. 22, 2018
[211] Morning Consult. What Americans Think About Marijuana in 2018, July 2018
[212] Melendez D. Baby boomers turning to cannabis instead of traditional pain meds. Las Vegas Now (Channel 8), November 16, 2018
[213] Cannabis Investing News. Understanding Customer Experience in the Cannabis Market. Investing News Network, November 25, 2018
[214] Bradford AC, Bradford WD. Medical Marijuana Laws Reduce Prescription Medication Use in Medicare Part D. Health Affairs, July 2016
[215] Bernberg M. MedMen: The Biggest Weed Company in the U.S. The Green Fund, November 6, 2018
[216] Pallardy C. Newly Public Lift & Co Looks to Accelerate Growth with More Data-Driven Products. New Cannabis Ventures, September 20, 2018
[217] JWT. High Times-from joints to a lifestyle movement: the rise of the cannabis economy, February 7, 2018
[218] Peltier D. Caribbean Destinations Gear Up for Pot Tourism Even While Weed Is Still Illegal. Skift, November 16, 2018
[219] Jordan K. Healthcare Is Becoming the New Retail. Forbes, June 23, 2017
[220] Credit Suisse. Apparel Retail & Brands: Making Sense of Softlines Following a Tumultuous Twelve Months, May 2017
[221] Nanos J. Dana-Farber to open clinic in Life Time Center. Boston Globe, June 12, 2017
[222] Rockett A. SRMC to expand services to medical mall at Biggs Park. The Robesonian, July 28, 2015
[223] JLL Research. Healthcare Real Estate Outlook, 2018
[224] Bachman R. Malls Never Wanted Gyms. Now They Court Them. Wall Street Journal, November 26, 2017
[225] Bachman R. Malls Never Wanted Gyms. Now They Court Them. Wall Street Journal, November 26, 2017
[226] Johnsen M. Hy-Vee partnership with Orangetheory Fitness a 'one-stop shop' for wellness. Drug Store News, August 31, 2017
[227] Edelman. Edelman Health Engagement Barometer, 2010
[228] IRI. Taking Charge: Consumers Grabbing Hold of Their Health and Wellness Drives $450-Billion Opportunity. November 2018
[229] IRi. 2017 Top Trends in Fresh Foods, September 2017
[230] Partnership for a Healthier America. 2018 Innovating a Healthier Future Summit, May 2-4, 2018. Presentation by Mike Lee, The Future of Food
[231] International Food Information Council Foundation. An Appetite for Health: Americans Over 50 Strive for Heart and Muscle Health, June 13 2018
[232] International Food Information Council Foundation. 2018 Food and Health Survey, May 16, 2018
[233] International Food Information Council Foundation. One-Third of Americans Are Dieting, Including One in 10 Who Fast – 2018 Food and Health Survey. May 16, 2018
[234] International Food Information Council Foundation. An Appetite for Health, June 2018
[235] Browne M. Grocery shopping has a hold on consumers, study finds. Supermarket News, June 26, 2018
[236] Food Marketing Institute. U.S. Grocery Shopper Trends 2018: The Shopper Desire to Eat Well and the Implications for Shopping, July 2018

[237] Sarasin L. The Symbiotic Relationship Between Eating Well And Shopping Well. Food Marketing Institute, August 15, 2018

[238] Gallagher E. Wal-Mart Supercenter opens in 'food desert' area. Chicago Tribune, May 31, 2016

[239] Hofbauer R. Kroger Launches Mobile App to Simplify, Score Healthy Eating. Progressive Grocer, July 16, 2018

[240] Keller, Megan E et al. "Enhancing Practice Efficiency and Patient Care by Sharing Electronic Health Records" Perspectives in health information management Vol. 12, Fall 1b. November 1, 2015

[241] Kroger press release. Kroger and GoodRx Launch the Kroger Rx Savings Club to Redefine the Customer Experience. December 12, 2018

[242] Patrick L, Dhruva SS, Shah ND, Ross JS. Medicare Beneficiary Out-of-Pocket Costs for Generic Cardiovascular Medications Available Through $4 Generic Drug Discount Programs. Annals of Internal Medicine, 4 December 2018

[243] Deloitte.

[244] Valinsky J. Aldi is going granola to compete with Whole Foods. CNN Money, August 16, 2018

[245] Retail Dietitian's Business Alliance. Coborn's Expands Their Supermarket Dietitian Program, September 14, 2016

[246] Redman R. Hy-Vee HealthMarket store makes debut. Supermarket News, August 3, 2018

[247] Ferguson T, with the e-Patients Scholars Working Group. e-Patients: how they can help us heal healthcare. Supported by Robert Wood Johnson Foundation Quality Health Care Grant #043806*

[248] Ferguson T. Online Health and the Empowered Medical Consumer. Presentation to Case Management Society of America, San Antonio, TX, June 27, 2003

[249] Rock Health. 50 things we now know about digital health consumers, December 13, 2016

[250] MacNeily A. Paging Dr. Google. Canadian Urological Association Journal, March-April 2013

[251] Rock Health. 50 Things We Now Know About Digital Health Consumers. December 13, 2016

[252] dotHealthLLC. Consumer Health Online – 2017 Research Report, October 2017

[253] Klick Health. 2017 Klick Health Consumer Survey on Healthcare Innovation, June 12, 2017

[254] Rock Health. Digital Health Consumer Adoption, 2015 261 Comscore. Cross-Platform Future in Focus U.S. 2017, March 2017

[255] Wireless Substitution: Early Release of Estimates from the National Health Interview Survey, July-December 2016.

[256] Comscore. 2017 U.S. Mobile App Report, August 24, 2017

[257] IQVIA. The Growing Value of Digital Health, November 2017

[258] Economist. Planet of the phones. February 26, 2015

[259] Fox BJ. Persuasive Technology: Using Computers to Change What We Think and Do. San Francisco CA: Morgan Kaufmann, December 2002

[260] IQVIA

[261] Pew Research Center. Americans' Views on Mobile Etiquette, August 26, 2015

[262] Ahonen TT. mAd Beyond Asia: How the Rest of the World Uses Mobile in Marketing. Mobile Marketing Association, MMA Forum, Singapore, August 22-23, 2013

[263] Brandis C. EHR Conversion and Smartphone Supported Wellness at Kaiser. Untethered Healthcare blog, December 16, 2009

[264] Accenture. Meet Today's Healthcare Team: Patients + Doctors + Machines – Accenture 2018 Consumer Survey on Digital Health, March 6, 2018

[265] Abt N. Smartphone apps help build a health community. Fleet Owner, November 14, 2018

[266] Accenture. Losing Patience: Why Healthcare Providers Need to Up Their Mobile Game, 2015

[267] Gent Edd. Smartphones can safeguard your health in some surprising ways. NBC News, January 2, 2018

[268] Bennett S. Wearables Could Catch Heart Problems That Elude Your Doctor. UCSF News Center, February 9. 2018

[269] Javelosa J, Reedy C. Giving up your smartphone could actually be bad for your health. Futurism, March 17, 2017

[270] Harris Interactive. Cell Pho

[271] American Journal of Managed Care. Interview with Dr. Joseph Kvedar, November 22, 2015. Accessed 30 November 2017 at:
http://www.ajmc.com/interviews/dr-joseph-kvedar-outlines-the-benefits-of-mobile-on-patient-engagement *

[272] Mann S. Research Shows Shortage of More than 100,000 Doctors by 2030. Association of American Medical Colleges (AAMC), March 14, 2017

[273] Ferguson T, with the e-Patients Scholars Working Group

[274] Sarasohn-Kahn J. Digital Health at CES 2017: Consumers Taking Health Into Their Own Hands. December 28, 2016

[275] IMS Health. Patient Adoption of mHealth: Use, Evidence and Remaining Barriers in Mainstream Acceptance. September 17, 2015

[276] McCracken H. HAPIfork: Can a Smart Utensil Make You a Smarter Eater? TIME, April 20, 2013

[277] Ibid.

[278] IQVIA Institute. The Growing Value of Digital Health – Evidence and Impact on Human Health and the Healthcare System. November 2017

[279] Forrester Research. Wearables Will Reach Critical-Mass Adoption by 2021. July 26, 2016

[280] IDC. Worldwide Wearables Market Grows 7.3% in Q3 2017 as Smart Wearables Rise and Basic Wearables Decline, Says IDC. November 30, 2017

[281] Martin C. Consumers Want Wearables for Health Fitness Info. MediaPost Connected Thinking, November 30, 2017

[282] Johnsen M. Getting on track with wearables. Drug Store News, December 13, 2017

[283] Sarasohn-Kahn J. Making Sense of Sensors: How New Technologies Can Change Patient Care. California HealthCare Foundation, February 2013

[284] Levi Strauss. The Type III Trucker Jacket Celebrates 50 Years. Unzipped Blog, October 2, 2017

[285] Yarns and Fibers News Bureau. Nanowear's SimplECG receives FDA nod, December 5, 2016

[286] Xue H, Westhues K, Joyce M, Leclerc O. Digital therapeutics: Preparing for take-off. McKinsey & Company, Februray 2018

[287] Novak, M. The Episode Where George Jetson Rages Against the Machine. Smithsonian, November 28, 2012

[288] Health Resources and Services Administration Federal Office of Rural Health Policy, U.S. Department of Health and Human Services. Accessed at:
http://www.hrsa.gov/ruralhealth/telehealth/

[289] PR Newswire. One in Five Consumers Would Switch to a Doctor that Offers Telehealth Visits, January 23, 2017

[290] Kaiser Family Foundation. 2018 Employer Health Benefits Survey, October 03, 2018

[291] National Business Group on Health. Large U.S. Employers Project Health Care Benefit Costs to Surpass $14,000 per Employee in 2018, National Business Group on Health Survey Finds. August 6, 2017

292 PR Newswire. "House Calls" Available at the Touch of a Button, April 4, 2017
293 Pearl RM. Engaging Physicians in Telehealth. NEJM Catalyst, March 29, 2016
294 Accenture. Voting for Virtual Health, February 9, 2017
295 Ibid.
296 Business Wire. Walgreens Introduces New Digital Marketplace Featuring 17 Leading Health Care Providers, July 26, 2018
297 RB press release. RB and Walmart Launch First-Of-Its-Kind Partnership with Doctor On Demand, Helping To Provide Healthcare Access To Consumers. October 17, 2018
298 BayCare press release. Walk-In Care Provided by BayCare Expands Access to Board-Certified Physicians, January 19, 2018
299 Higi Press Release. higi Launches Groundbreaking Population Screening Solution for Healthcare Businesses, February 19. 2017
300 Salazar D. New higi partnership opens doors to patient data. Drug Store News, December 4, 2018
301 Kantar Millward Brown. 2017 BrandZ Global Top 100, June 2017
302 Tibken S. Apple's Tim Cook dishes on taxes and the demise of money. CNET, 13 February 2018
303 Apple website accessed on February 13, 2018 at: https://www.apple.com/healthcare/
304 Apple newsroom. Apple announces effortless solution bringing health records to iPhone, January 24, 2018, press release
305 Farr C, Sullivan M. Apple Acquires Personal Health Data Startup Gliimpse. Fast Company, August 22, 2016
306 Apple. Doctors put patients in charge with Apple's Health Records feature. Press release, March 29, 2018
307 Stanford Medicine News Center. Stanford launches smartphone app to study heart health, March 9, 2015
308 Cortez MF, Chen C. Thousands Have Already Signed Up for Apple's ResearchKit. Bloomberg Technology, March 11, 2015
309 Krishnan N. Apple in Healthcare. CBInsights, November 2018
310 Ritchie R. Apple Health: The Next Big Thing. iMore, December 5, 2018
311 Metz R. CES 2015: The Internet of Just About Everything. MIT Technology Review, January 6, 2016
312 BabyCenter. 71 Percent of Today's Parents Own at Leaset One 'Internet of Things' Device & Three-Quarters of Those Without IoT are Interested and Want to Learn More, According to BabyCenter Research. Press release, January 4, 2017
313 Kvedar J. The Internet of Healthy Things. Boston, MA: Partners Connected Health, 2015
314 Fox S and Duggan M. Tracking for Health. Pew Research Center, January 28, 2013
315 Centers for Disease Control and Prevention. Health, United States, 2016, Table 53
316 Guy GP, Thomas CC, Thompson T, Watson M, Massetti GM, Richardson LC. Vital signs: Melanoma incidence and mortality trends and projections—United States, 1982–2030. Morbidity & Mortality Weekly Report. 2015;64(21):591-596
317 Rogers HW, Weinstock MA, Feldman SR, Coldiron BM. Incidence estimate of nonmelanoma skin cancer (keratinocyte carcinomas) in the US population. JAMA Dermatology, April 30, 2015
318 Stern, RS. Prevalence of a history of skin cancer in 2007: results of an incidence-based model. Archives of Dermatology, 2010; 146(3):279-282
319 Cavoukian A. Privacy by Design: The 7 Foundational Principles. Information and Privacy Commissioner of Ontario, revised January 2011
320 Ranft F, Adler M, Diamond P, Guerrero E, Laza M. Policy Network. Freeing the Road: Shaping the future for autonomous vehicles. Policy Network, November 2016

321 Wayland M. FCA plans to produce Chrysler Portal concept after 2018. The Detroit News, January 11, 2017

322 Wilson M. Who Needs a Hospital When This Self Driving Doctor Comes to You? Fast Company Design, June 21, 2017

323 Hsiao C-J, Hing E. Use and Characteristics of Electronic Health Record Systems Among Office-based Physician Practices: United States, 2001-2013. U.S. Department of Health and Human Services, Centers for Disease Control and Prevention, national center for health Statistics. NCHS Data Brief, No. 143, January2 014

324 Office of the National Coordinator for Health Information Technologiy. Hospital Progress to Meaningful Use by Size, Type, and Urban/Rural Location, August 2017

325 Office of the National Coordinator for Health Information Technology. Percent of REC Enrolled Providers by Practice Type Live on an HER and Demonstrating Meaningful Use, January 2016

326 Center for Health Transformation, Merritt D (ed.). Paper Kills - Transforming Health and Healthcare with Information Technology. Washington DC: CHT Press, June 5, 2007

327 Sternstein A. Gingrich: 'Paper kills,' electronic medical records save lives. Healthcare IT News, September 16, 2005

328 Committee on Quality of Health Care in America, Institute of Medicine. Crossing the Quality Chasm: A New Health System for the 21st Century. Washington DC: National Academy Press, July 2001

329 Fry E, Schulte F. Death by a Thousand Clicks: Where Electronic Health Records Went Wrong. Fortune and Kaiser Health News, March 18, 2019

330ECRI Institute. 2019 Top 10 Patient Safety Concerns, March 11, 2019

331 Woods SS, Schwartz E, Tuepker A, Press NA, Nazi KM, Nichol WP, Turvey, CL. Patient Experiences With Full Electronic Access to Health Records and Clinical Notes Through My HealtheVet Personal Health Record Pilot: Qualitative Study. Journal of Medical Internet Research, Vol 15, No 3 (2013): March

332 California Healthcare Foundation. Consumers and Health Information Technology: A National Survey, April 2010

333 Zurovac J, Dale S, Kovac M. Perceptions of Electronic Health Records and Their Effect on the Quality of Care: Resutls from a Survey of Patients in Four States. Mathematica Policy Research, November 2012

334 Quinn MA, Kats AM, Kleinman K, Bates DW, Simon SR. The Relationship Between Electronic Health Records and Malpractice Claims. JAMA Archives of Internal Medicine. August 13/27. 2012, Vol 172, No 15

335 Delbanco T, Walker J, Darer JD, Elmore JG, Feldman HJ, Leveille SG, et al. Open Notes: Doctors and Patients Signing On. Annals of Internal Medicine;153:121–125, July 20, 2010

336 Sadick B. New System Makes it Easier for Patients to Talk to Doctors. Wall Street Journal, February 25, 2018

337 Brohan M. Four big hospitals will give active voice to passive online doc notes. Internet Health Management, November 17, 2017

338 Rock Health. Healthcare consumers in a digital transition, September 2018

339 Alston C, Paget L, Halvorson G, Novelli B, Guest J, McCabe P, Hoffman K, Koepke C, Simon M, Sutton S, Okun S, Wicks P, Undem T, Rohrbach V, Von Kohorn I. Communicating with Patients on Health Care Evidence. Institute of Medicine of the National Academies, September 2012

340 PatientsLikeMe press release. PatientsLikeMe Launches "Data for Good" Campaign to Encourage Health Data Sharing to Advance Medicine, March 10, 2014

341 Betts D, Korenda L. Inside the patient journey: Three key touch points for consumer engagement strategies. Findings form the Deloitte 2018 Health Care Consumer Survey. September 25, 2018

[342] Johnsen M. Walgreens app makes health tracking easy. Drug Store News, December 13, 2017

[343] Fox S. The Network is Our Superpower. Susannah Fox Blog, January 20, 2014

[344] Morris M. Margaret Morris: The new sharing of emotions, TED Talk, May 6, 2013

[345] Hoch D, Ferguson T. What I've learned from E-patients. PLoS Med. 2005;2(8):e206.

[346] FY2015 Annual Report, Patient-Centered Outcomes Research Institute, October 1, 2014 – September 30, 2015

[347] Accenture Consulting. Accenture 2016 Consumer Survey on Patient Engagement, June 29, 2016

[348] Gardner C. Med Center Health security breach addressed. WBKO (ABC13), March 29, 2017

[349] Protenus, Inc. Q3 2018 Breach Barometer: Insider-wrongdoing accounts for increasing number of breached patient records over the course of 2018. November 2018

[350] Beazley. Beazley 2018 Breach Briefing, February 20, 2018

[351] Ponemon Institute and IBM Security, The 2018 Cost of a Data Breach Study, June 2018

[352] Data Guardian. The Definitive Guide to DLP – Healthcare Edition, July 28, 2017

[353] Verizon, 2017 Breach Report, April 27, 2017

[354] Protenus 368 Rashid FY. Why hackers want your health care data most of all. InfoWorld, September 14, 2015

[355] Wollan R, Barton R, Ishikawa M, Quiring K. Put Your Trust in Hyper-Relevance. Accenture, January 15, 2018

[356] Mallonee MK, Scott E. Comey: "There is no such thing as absolute privacy in America." CNN, March 9, 2017

[357] Sprenger P. Sun on Privacy: "Get Over It." Wired, January 26, 1999

[358] Olmstead K, Smith A. Many Americans do not trust modern institutions to protect their personal data – even as they frequently neglect cybersecurity best practices in their own personal lives. Pew Research Center, January 26, 2017

[359] Soergel A. Equifax Breach Could Have 'Decades of Impact." US News & World Report, September 8, 2017

[360] Fowler B. Americans Want More Say in the Privacy of Personal Data. Consumer Reports, May 18, 2017

[361] Rainie L. The state of privacy in post-Snowden America. Pew Research Center, September 21, 2016

[362] Morey T, Forbath T, Schoop A. Customer Data: Designing for Transparency and Trust. Harvard Business Review, May 2015

[363] Kirzinger A, Sugarman E, Wu B, Brodie M. Kaiser Health Tracking Poll: August 2016. Kaiser Family Foundation, September 1, 2016

[364] Rainie L, Duggan M. Privacy and Information Sharing. Pew Research Center, January 14, 2016

[365] Mack H. Thirty-six connected health apps and devices the FDA cleared in 2016. MobiHealthNews, December 30, 2016

[366] MobiHealthNews. Fifty-one connected health products the FDA cleared in 2017. December 21, 2017

[367] Sarasohn-Kahn J. Here's Looking at You: How Personal Health Information Is Being Tracked and Used. California Healthcare Foundation, July 2014

[368] Singer N. How Companies Scour Our Digital Lives for Clues to Our Health. New York Times, February 25, 2018

[369] Jain SH, Powers BW, Hawkins JB, Brownstein JS. The digital phenotype. Nature Biotechnology, May 2015

[370] Freifeld CC, Mandl KD, Reis BY, Brownstein JS. HealthMap: Global Infectious Disease Monitoring through Automated Classification and Visualization of

Internet Media Reports. Journal of the AMIA 2008 Mar- Apr; 15(2):150-157

[371] Rosati KB. HIPAA privacy: the compliance challenges ahead. Journal of Health Law. 2002 Winter; 35(1):45-82

[372] Office of the National Coordinator, U.S. Department of Health and Human Services. Examining Oversight of the Privacy & Security of Health Data Collected by Entities Not Regulated by HIPAA. June 17, 2016

[373] Neff G, Nafus D. Self-Tracking. Cambridge, MA: MIT Press, June 2016

[374] Partridge SR, Gallagher P, Freeman B, Gallagher R. Facebook Groups for the Management of Chronic Diseases. Journal of Medical Internet Research, January 2018 vol. 20, issue 1

[375] Dhar VK, Kim Y, Graff JT, Jung AD, Garrett J, Dick LE, Harris J, Shah SA. Benefit of social media on patient engagement and satisfaction: Result of a 9-month, qualitative pilot study using Facebook. Surgery, March 2018 Vol 163, Issue 3

[376] Hickman B. How We Used Facebook to Power Our Investigation Into Patient Harm. ProPublica, December 19, 2012

[377] Lupton D. Digital Health: Critical and Cross-Disciplinary Perspectives. London and New York: Routledge, August 30, 2017

[378] Duhigg C. How Companies Learn Your Secrets. New York Times, February 16, 2012

[379] Deloitte. 2017 Global Mobile Consumer Survey – US edition – The dawn of the next era in mobile, 2017

[380] Kroft S. The Data Brokers. 60 Minutes, March 9, 2014

[381] Hsiao C-J, Hing E, Socey TC, Cai B. Electronic Medical Record/Electronic Health Record Systems of Office-based Physicians: United States: 2009 and Preliminary 2010 State Estimates. National Center for Health Statistics, Centers for Disease Control, U.S. Department of Health and Human Services, December 2010

[382] IQVIA Institute. The Growing Value of Digital Health: Evidence and Impact on Human Health and the Healthcare System, November 2017

[383] Ackerman L. Mobile Health and Fitness Applications and Information Privacy: Report to California Consumer Protection Foundation. Privacy Rights Clearinghouse, July 15, 2013

[384] The American Presidency Project. Statement on Signing the Health Insurance Portability and Accountability Act of 1996, August 21, 1996

[385] Snell E. How Do HIPAA Regulations Apply to Wearable Devices? Health IT Security, March 23, 2017

[386] Singer N. An American Quilt of Privacy Laws, Incomplete. The New York Times, March 30, 2013

[387] Sharma C. US Mobile Market Update 2017. Chetan Sharma Consulting, February 20, 2018

[388] Gitlin JM. Connected cars are going to monetize data, but most drivers don't know that. Ars Technica, February 22, 2018

[389] Foley & Lardner LLP. 2017 Connected Cars & Autonomous Vehicles Survey, October 24, 2017

[390] Alliance of Automobile Manufacturers. Automotive Industry Collaborates in Developing Vehicle Cybersecurity Best Practices to Address Cybersecurity Challenges. July 21, 2016

[391] The White House, Office of the Press Secretary. President Policy Directive – Critical Infrastructure Security and Resilience, PPD-21, February 12, 2013

[392] U.S. Government Accountability Office. Vehicle Data Privacy: Industry and Federal Efforts Under Way but NHTSA Needs to Define Its Role. GAO-17-656, July 28, 2017

[393] Coppola G, Welch D. The Car of the Future Will Sell Your Data. Bloomberg, February 20, 2018

[394] O'Connor N. Reforming the U.S. Approach to Data Protection and Privacy. Council on Foreign Relations, January 30, 2018

[395] Standen A. Patient's Crusade for Access to their Medical Device Data. KQED, May 28, 2012

[396] Versel N. Twitter helps data liberation advocate Campos to a small victory. MobiHealthNews, July 30, 2013

[397] Neff G, Nafus D. Self-Tracking. Cambridge MA: The MIT Press, June 24, 2016

[398] Pittman D. Cancer moonshot head recounts exchange with Epic's Faulkner. Politico, August 2, 2017

[399] Chetty R, Stepner M, Abraham S, Lin S, Scuderi B, Turner N, Bergeron A, Cutler D. The Association Between Income and Life Expectancy in the United States, 2001-2014. JAMA 2016;315(16):1750-1766, April 2016

[400] World Health Organization

[401] McGinnis JM, Foege WJ. Actual Causes of Death in the United States. JAMA, November 10, 1993, Vol, 270, No. 18

[402] McKeown T. The Role of Medicine: Dream, Mirage, or Nemesis? London: Nuffield Provincial Hospitals Trust, 1976

[403] Parks T. Death by ZIP Code: Investigating the root causes of health inequity. AMA Wire, August 25, 2016

[404] Erreygers G, Kessels R. Socioeconomic Status and Health: A New Approach to the Measurement of Bivariate Inequality. International Journal of Environmental Research and Public Health. July 2017;14(7):673

[405] Martinson ML, Reichman NE. Socioeconomic Inequalities in Low Birth Weight in the United States, the United Kingdom, Canada, and Australia. American Journal of Public Health. 2016;106(4):748-54

[406] Adler NE, Newman K. Socioeconomic disparities in health: pathways and Policies. Health Affairs, Volume 21, Number 2, March/April 2002

[407] Feinstein, J. (1993). The Relationship between Socioeconomic Status and Health: A Review of the Literature. The Milbank Quarterly, 71(2), 279-322

[408] Martinson ML, Reichman NE. Socioeconomic Inequalities in Low Birth Weight in the United States, the United Kingdom, Canada, and Australia. American Journal of Public Health, Vol. 105, No. 4, April 2016

[409] Adler

[410] Kaplan RM, Spittel ML, David DH. Population Health: Behavioral and Social Science Insights. Agency for Healthcare Research and Quality, July 2015

[411] Olshansky SJ, Antonucci T, Berkman L, Binstock R, et al. Differences in Life Expectancy Due to Race and Educational Differences Are Widening, And Many May Not Catch Up. Health Affairs 31, No. 8 (2012): 1803-1813

[412] Accenture. The Hidden Cost of Healthcare System Complexity, September 12, 2018

[413] Mohr, GB. The changing significance of different stressors after the announcement of bankruptcy: A longitudinal investigation with special emphasis on job insecurity. Journal of Organizational Behavior 23, 337-359, April 12, 2000

[414] Sverke M, Hellgren J, Näswall K. No security: a meta-analysis and review of job insecurity and its consequences. Journal of Occupational Health Psychology 2002 Jul;7(3):242-64

[415] Heaney, CA, Israel BA, House JS. Chronic job insecurity among automobile workers: Effects on job satisfaction and health. Social Science & Medicine 38(10): 1431-1437, May 1994

[416] Longhi S, Nandi A, Bryan M, Connolly S, Gedikli C. Gender and unemployment. Analysis of Understanding Society: the UK Household Longitudinal Survey. What Works Wellbeing Centre, October 2017

[417] Perissinotto CM, Cenzer IS, Covinsky KE. Loneliness in Older Persons: A predictor of functional decline and death. Archives of Internal Medicine. 2012 July 23; 172(14):1078-1083

[418] Wilson RS, Krueger KR, Arnold SE, et al. Loneliness and Risk of Alzheimer Disease. Archives of General Psychiatry. 2007;64(2):234-240

[419] Valtorta NK, Kanaan M, Gilbody S, et al. Loneliness and social isolation as risk

factors for coronary heart disease and stroke: systematic review and meta-analysis of longitudinal observational studies. Heart 2016;102:1009-1016

[420] Nicholson NR. A review of social isolation: an important but under-assessed condition in older adults. Journal of Primary Prevention 2012 Jun;33(2-3):137-52

[421] Alcaraz KI, Eddens KS, Blasé JL, Diver WR, et al. Social Isolation and Mortality in US Black and White Men and Women. American Journal of Epidemiology, 16 October 2018

[422] Flowers L, Houser A, Noel-Miller C, et al. Medicare Spends More on Socially Isolated Adults. AARP Public Policy Institute, November 2017

[423] Coleman-Jensen A, Rabbitt MP, Gregory CA, Singh A. Household Food Security in the United States in 2017. United States Department of Agriculture, September 2018

[424] Gundersen C, Ziliak JP. Food Insecurity and Health Outcomes. Health Affairs. 34 No. 11 (2015): 1830-1939, November 2015

[425] Zaliak, J. P., Gundersen, C. The health consequences of senior hunger in the United States: Evidence from the 1999-2010 NHANES. National Foundation to End Senior Hunger, February 2014

[426] Berkowitz, Seth A.; Seligman, Hilary K.; and Basu, Sanjay, "Impact of Food Insecurity and SNAP Participation on Healthcare Utilization and Expenditures" (2017). University of Kentucky Center for Poverty Research Discussion Paper Series. 103

[427] Swinburne M, Garfield K, Wasserman AR. Reducing Hospital Readmissions: Addressing the Impact of Food Security and Nutrition. Law and Medical Ethics. 2017 Mar;45(1_suppl):86-89

[428] Slopen N, Fitzmaurice G, Williams DR, Gilman SE. Poverty, Food Insecurity, and the Behavior for Childhood Internalizing and Externalizing Disorders. Journal of the American Academy of Child U& Adolescent Psychiatry, Volume 49, Number 5, May 2010

[429] Leung CW, Epel ES, Willett WC, Rimm EB, Laraia BA. Household Food Insecurity Is Positively Associated with Depression among Low-Income Supplemental Nutrition Assistance Program Participants and Income-Eligible Nonparticipants. The Journal of Nutrition 2015 March;145(3):622-7

[430] Syed ST, Gerber BS, Sharp LK. Traveling Towards Disease: Transportation Barriers to Health care Access. Journal of Community Health 2013 October;38(5):976-993

[431] Syed ST, Gerber BS, Sharp LK. Traveling towards disease: transportation barriers to health care access. Journal of Community Health. 2013 October;38(5):976-93

[432] American Public Health Association and the Safe Routes to School National Partnership. Fighting for Equitable Transportation: Why It Matters, 2015

[433] U.S. Department of Health and Human Services, Office of the Surgeon General. The Health Consequences of Smoking – 50 Years of Progress: A Report of the Surgeon General, 2014

[434] Greenstone M, Fan CQ. Introducing the Air Quality Life Index. Energy Policy Institute at the University of Chicago, November, 2018

[435] The Lancet Commission on pollution and health. The Lancet, Vol, 301, No. 10119, October 19, 2017

[436] Zhang Y, et al. Long-term trends in the ambient PM2.5- and O3-related mortality burdens in the United States under emission reductions from 1990 to 2010 . Atmospheric Chemistry and Physics 18, 15003-15016, 2018

[437] Philip A, Sims E, Houston J, Konieczny R. 63 million Americans exposed to unsafe drinking water. USA Today, August 14, 2017

[438] American Society of Civil Engineers. 2017 Infrastructure Report Card, March 9, 2017

[439] U.S. Environmental Protection Agency. Overview of Water-related Diseases and Contaminants in Private Wells. Accessed from

https://www.epa.gov/privatewells/potential-well-water-contaminants-and-their-impacts on 29 November 2018
[440] U.S. Global Change Research Program. Fourth National Climate Assessment, November 23, 2018
[441] National Center of Healthy Housing, Healthy Homes Principles
[442] Centers for Disease Control. Prevention Tips (Lead). Accessed 3 December 2018 at: https://www.cdc.gov/nceh/lead/tips.htm
[443] Hood CM, Gennuso KP, Swain GR, Catlin BB. County Health Rankings: Relationships Between Determinant Factors and Health Outcomes. American Journal of Preventive Medicine 2016 Feb;50(2):129-35
[444] Milliman M, editor. Access to health care in America. Institute of Medicine (US) Committee on Monitoring Access to Personal Health Care. Washington (DC): National Academies Press, 1993.
[445] Cain MC, Sarasohn-Kahn J, Wayne JC. Health e-People: The Online Consumer Experience. Institute for the Future, August 2000
[446] Sternberg PL. Rural Individuals' Telehealth Practices: An Overview. United States Department of Agriculture, Economic Research Service, November 2018
[447] AMIA. Letter to Ajit Pai, Commission of the FCC, RE: Request for Comment-Actions to Accelerate Adoption and accessibility of Broadband-Enabled Health Care Solutions and Advanced Technologies (GN Docket No. 16-46, FCC 17-46), May 24, 2017
[448] FCC. Request for Comment and Data on Actions to Accelerate Adoption and Accessibility of Broadband-Enabled Health Care Solutions and Advanced Technologies, 82 FR 21781 (May 10, 2017). Federal Register: The Daily Journal of the United States
[449] Sarasohn-Kahn J. Broadband Connectivity Is a Social Determinant of Health. Huffington Post, July 22, 2016
[450] Blue Cross Blue Shield Association. The Health of America Report: Understanding Health Conditions Across the U.S. December 14, 2017
[451] Gallup-Sharecare Well-Being Index. State of American Well-Being: The Cost of Diabetes in the U.S.: Economic and Well-Being Impact, November 13, 2018
[452] Pruitt Z, Emechebe N, Quast T, Taylor P, Bryant K. Expenditure Reductions Associated with a Social Service Referral Program. Population Health Management, 17 April 2018
[453] McKeown
[454] Daniel H, Bornstein SS, Kane GC, for the Health and Public Policy Committee of the American College of Physicians. Addressing Social Determinants to Improve Patient Care and Promote Health Equity: An American College of Physicians Position Paper. Annals of Internal Medicine, April 17, 2018
[455] Wesleyan Median Project. 2018: The Health Care Election. October 18. 2018
[456] Collins SR, Gunja MZ, Doty MM, Bhupal HK. Americans' Views on Health Insurance at the End of a Turbulent Year. Commonwealth Fund, M1, 2018
[457] Stein L, Cornwell S, Tanfani J. Inside the progressive movement roiling the Democratic Party. Reuters, August 23, 2018
[458] Kliff S. They're on Obamacare, they voted for Trump, and they're already disappointed, Vox, June 7, 2017
[459] McCarthy J. Six in 10 Americans Worry About Higher Healthcare Premiums. Gallup, December 10, 2018
[460] Newport F. Government Favored to Ensure Healthcare – Just Not Deliver It. Gallup, December 3, 2018
[461] Bauchner H. Health Care in the United States: A Right or a Privilege? JAMA, January 3, 2017
[462] Tyson P. The Hippocratic Oath Today. NOVA, WHYY, March 27, 2001
[463] Tsiompanou E, Marketos SG. Hippocrates: timeless still. Journal of the Royal Society of Medicine. 2013 Jul; 106(7):288-292
[464] Robinson J. The Oxford Companion to Wine. New York: Oxford University Press, 2006

465 Macintyre S, Ellaway A. Neighbourhoods and Health: Overview, in Neighbourhoods and Health, Kawachi I, Berkman L eds. New York: Oxford University Press, 2003

466 Kish G. A Source Book in Geography. Cambridge MA: Harvard University Press, 1978

467 Zahran, Sammy et al. Four phases of the Flint Water Crisis: Evidence from blood lead levels in children. Environmental Research Vol. 157 (2017)

468 Lanphear BP, Rauch S, Auinger P, Allen RW, Hornung RW. Low-level lead exposure and mortality in US adults: a population-based cohort study. The Lancet Volume 3, Issue 4, April 1, 2018

469 Cuthbertson, Courtney A et al. Angry, Scared, and Unsure: Mental Health Consequences of Contaminated Water in Flint, Michigan. Journal of Urban Health – Bulletin of the New York Academy of Medicine Vol. 93,6 (2016)

470 Temkin O, In Early History. In Social Medicine: Its Derivatives and Objectives. Galdston I, ed., New York: The Commonwealth Fund, 1949

471 Tountas Y. The historical origins of the basic concepts of health promotion and education: the role of ancient Greek philosophy and medicine. Health Promotion International, Vol. 24, Issue 2, June 2009

472 Ariely D. The 2009 TIME 100: Nicholas Christakis. TIME, April 30, 2009

473 Christakis N, Fowler J. Connected: The Surprising Power of Our Social Networks and How They Shape Our Lives. Little, Brown, 2009

474 Smith KP, Christakis NA. Social Networks and Health. Annual Review of Sociology, March 24, 2008

475 Berkman LF, Syme SL. Social networks, host-resistance, and mortality – 9-year follow-up study of Alameda County residents. American Journal of Epidemiology, February 1979. Cassel J. Contribution of social-environment to host-resistance – 4th Wade Hampton Frost Lecture. American Journal of Epidemiology, August 1976. Cobb S. Social support as a moderator of life stress. Psychosomatic Medicine, September-October 1976

476 Steptoe A, Shankar A, Demakakos P, Wardle J. Social isolation, loneliness, and all-0cause mortality in older men and women. Proceedings of the National Academy of Science, April 9. 2013

477 Jain SH. The Growing Imperative to Address Senior Loneliness. NEJM Catalyst February 27, 2018

478 Yang YC, Boen C, Gerken K, Li T, Schorpp K, Mullan Harris K. Social relationships and physiological determinants of longevity across the human life span. Proceedings of the National Academy of Science, January 19, 2016

479 Christakis

480 Cacioppo JT, Fowler JH, Christakis NA. Alone in the Crowd: The Structure and Spread of Loneliness in a Large Social Network. Journal of Personality and Social Psychology, December 2009

481 Inspired by Putnam R. Bowling Alone. Simon & Schuster (Touchstone Books), 2001

482 Krueger PM, Tran MK, Hummer RA, Chang VW. Mortality Attributable to Low Levels of Education in the United States. PLOS One, July 8, 2015

483 Felitti VJ, Anda RF, Nordenberg D, Williamson DF, et al. Relationship of Childhood Abuse and Household Dysfunction to Many of the Leading Causes of Death in Adults – The Adverse Childhood Experiences (ACE) Study, American Journal of Preventive Medicine 1998;14(4)

484 Centers for Disease Control. Adverse Childhood Experience Journal Articles by Topic Area. Website accessed 20 December 2018 at: https://www.cdc.gov/violenceprevention/acestudy/journal.html

485 Pollack CE, Cubbin C, Sania A, Hayward M, Vallone D, Flaherty B, Braveman PA. Do Wealth Disparities Contribute to Health Disparities within Racial/Ethnic Groups? Journal of Epidemiology and Community Health 67 (5): 439–45, 2013

486 Woolf SH, Aron L, Dubay L, Luk KX, Zimmerman E, Simon SM. How Are

Income and Wealth Linked to Health and Longevity. Urban Institute, April 2015
[487] Case A, Deaton A. Mortality and Morbidity in the 21st Century. Brookings Institution, March 23, 2017
[488] Belluz J. Why the white middle class is dying faster, explained in 6 charts. Vox, May 23, 2017
[489] The World Bank, National Accounts Data, 2017. Accessed December 18, 2018 at: https://data.worldbank.org/indicator/NY.GDP.MKTP.CD
[490] Kochhar R, Fru R, Rohal M. Pew Research Center, December 9, 2015
[491] SHADAC. Fifty-State Analysis Finds Lower Access to Care among Adults with Less Education. Press release, March 21, 2018
[492] Braveman P, Egerter S, Barclay C. Income, Wealth and Health, Exploring the Social Determinants of Health. Robert Wood Johnson Foundation, 2011
[493] St. John A. How the Affordable Care Act Drove Down Personal Bankruptcy. Consumer Reports, May 2, 2017
[494] Austin DA. Medical Debt as a Cause of Consumer Bankruptcy. Maine Law Review, 2014
[495] Emerson RW. The Conduct of Life, 1860
[496] Alley DE, Lloyd J, Shardell M, Pagan JA, Pollack CE, Cannuscio C. Mortgage Delinquency and Changes in Access to Health Resources and Depressive Symptoms in a Nationally Representative Cohort of Americans Older Than 50 Years. American Journal of Public Health, December 2011
[497] Stuckler D, Basu S. The Body Economic: Why Austerity Kills. Basic Books, May 21, 2013
[498] Cuckler GA, SIsko AM, Poisal JA, Keehan SP, Smith SD, Madison AJ, Wolfe CJ, Hardesty JC. National Health Expenditure Projections, 2017-26: Despite Uncertainty, Fundamentals Primarily Drive Spending Growth. Health Affairs, February 14, 2018
[499] TransAmerica Center for Health Studies. Healthcare Consumers in a Time of Uncertainty: Fifth Annual Nationwide TCHS Survey, October 2017
[500] Gallup. Americans Still Hold Dim View of U.S. Healthcare System, December 11, 2017
[501] Gallup. Confidence in Institutions, accessed at: http://news.gallup.com/poll/1597/confidence-institutions.aspx
[502] Chubb.The 2018 Chubb Cyber Risk Survey, September 25, 2018
[503] Nakagawa K, Kvedar J, Yellowlees P. Retail Outlets Using Telehealth Pose Significant Policy Questions for Health Care. Health Affairs, 37, No, 12 (2018)
[504] Stanford Medicine. 2018 Health Trends Report: The Democratization of Health Care, December 2018
[505] Deloitte. First control, then consent, September 6, 2018. Data point from Digital Media Trends Survey: A New World of Choice for Digital Consumers, Deloitte Insights, March 19, 2018
[506] European Data Protection Supervisor, European Union. Meeting the challenges of big data. Opinion7/2015, 19 November 2015
[507] De La Torre L. GDPR matchup: The California Consumer Privacy Act 2018. International Association of Privacy Professionals, July 31, 2018
[508] Mikk K, Sleeper HA, Topol EJ. The Pathway to Patient Data Ownership and Better Health. JAMA, October 17, 2017
[509] Tanner A. Our Bodies, Our Data. Boston, MA: Beacon Press, 2017
[510] Fisher N, Carges J. Your Health Records Don't Belong to You. It's Time You Demand Them! Forbes, November 27, 2017
[511] Tanner A. How Data Brokers Make Money Off Your Medical Records. Scientific American, February 1, 2016
[512] Topol E. The Patient Will See You Now. New York: Basic Books, 2016
[513] Campos C, Sebastian A. Data liberación: The Path to Precision Medicine. The White House blog, July 9, 2015
[514] Robbins G. Need a little extra money? You'll soon be able to sell and rent your

DNA. San Diego Union-Tribune, June 5, 2018

[515] Molteni M. Ancestry's Genetic Testing Kits Are Heading for Your Stocking This Year. Wired, December 1, 2017

[516] Beeman RR. Perspectives on the Constitution: A Republic, If You Can Keep It. National Constitution Center, Philadelphia

[517] Allen D. Is affordable health care a basic right? Believe it or not, Republicans think so. Washington Post, January 12 2017

[518] Miles E. Self-Health as a Habit. New York: EP Dutton & Company, 1919

[519] Waples EJ. Self-Health: The Politics of Care in American Literature, 1793-1873. Dissertation submitted for PhD, The University of Michigan, 2016